NURSING HISTORY REVIEW

VOLUME 15–2007

D1617172

NURSING HISTORY REVIEW

Patricia D'Antonio, Editor
Barbra Mann Wall, Book Review Editor
Elizabeth Weiss, Assistant Editor

Editorial Review Board

Ellen D. Baer
Florida

Susan Baird
Pennsylvania

Nettie Birnbach
Florida

Eleanor Crowder Bjoring
Texas

Barbara Brodie
Virginia

Olga Maranjian Church
Connecticut

Donna Diers
Connecticut

Julie Fairman
Pennsylvania

Marilyn Flood
California

Janet Golden
New Jersey

Diane Hamilton
Michigan

Carol Helmstadter
Ontario, Canada

Wanda C. Hiestand
New York

Joan Lynaugh
Pennsylvania

Lois Monteiro
Rhode Island

Siobon Nelson
Toronto, Canada

John Parascandola
Maryland

Anne-Marie Rafferty
London, United Kingdom

Susan Reverby
Massachusetts

Naomi Rogers
Connecticut

Nancy Tomes
New York

NURSING HISTORY REVIEW

OFFICIAL PUBLICATION OF THE
AMERICAN ASSOCIATION FOR THE HISTORY OF NURSING

1062-8061   2007 – Volume 15

CONTENTS

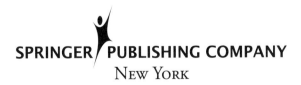

SPRINGER PUBLISHING COMPANY
NEW YORK

Cover Photo: A Wisconsin nurse weighing a baby in the 1930s. Reprinted courtesy
of the Wisconsin Historical Society.

Nursing History Review is published annually for the American Association for the History of Nursing Inc., by Springer Publishing Company, LLC, New York.

Business office: All business correspondence, including subscriptions, renewals, advertising, and address changes, should be sent to Springer Publishing Company, LLC, 11 West 42nd Street, New York, NY 10036.

Editorial officer: Submissions and editorial correspondance should be directed to Parricia D'Antonio, Editor, *Nursing History Review,* University of Pennsylvania, 420 Guardian Drive, Room 307, Philadelphia, PA 19104–6096. See *Guidelines for contributors* on page ix for further details.

Members of the American Association for the History of Nursing, Inc. (AAHN) receive *Nursing History Review* on payment of annual membership dues. Applications and other correspondance relating to AAHN membership should be directed to: Janet L Fickeissen, Executive Secretary, American Association for the History of Nursing, Inc., P. O. Box 175, Lonoka Harbor, NJ 08734–0175.

Subscription rates: Volume 15, 2007. For institutions: $85/1 year, $150/2 year. For individulas; $45/1 year, $80/2 years. Outside the United States—For institutions: $95/1 year, $170/2 years: for individuals: $55/1 year, $90/2 years. Air shipment is available for an additional $12/year. Payment must be made in advance by check (in U.S. dollars drawn on a US bank) or international money order, payable to Springer Publishing Company, LLC, or by MasterCard, Visa, or American Express.

Indexes/abstracts of articles appear in: CINAHL® print index & database, Current Contents/ Social & Behavioral Science, Social Sciences Citation Index, Research Alert, RNdex, Index Medicus/MEDLINE, History Abstracts, America; History and Life.

Permission: All rights are reserved. No part of this volume may be reproduced or utilized in any form or by any means, electronic or mechanical, including photocopying (with the exception listed below), recording, or by any information storage and retrievel system, without permission in writing from the publisher. Permission is granted by the copyright owner for libraries and others registered with the Copyright Clearance Center (CCC) to photocopy any artical herein for $5,00 per copy of the article. Payments should be sent directly to Copyright Clearence Center, 27 Congress Street, Salem, MA 01970, U.S.A. This permission holds for copying done for personal or internal reference use only: it does not extend to other kinds of copying, such as copying for general distribution, advertising or promotional purposes, creating new collective works, or for resale. Requests for these permissions or further information should be addressed to Springer Publishing Company, LLC.

Postmaster: Send address change to Springer Publishing Company, LCC, 11 West 42nd Street, New York, NY 10036.

Copyright © 2007 by Springer Publishing Company, LCC New York, for the American Association for the History of Nursing, Inc. Printed in the United States of America on acid-free paper.

ISSN 1062–8061   ISBN 0–8261–1483–0

Printed in the United States by Bang Printing

GUIDELINES FOR CONTRIBUTORS

The *Nursing History Review,* the official publication of the American Association for the History of Nursing, is peer-reviewed and published annually for subscribers and members of the Association. Original research manuscripts are welcomed in broad areas related to the history of nursing, health care, health policy, and society. The *Review* prefers manuscripts of approximately 40 pages, inclusive of endnotes.

Submitted manuscripts must be prepared using the guidelines specified in the *Chicago Manual of Style,* 15th edition. Manuscripts must have a title page that contains the full title of the manuscript, the author(s) name(s) as they are meant to appear in print, institutional affiliations and preferred mailing addresses <u>for all authors</u>, and relevant contact information for the corresponding author. The title page also lists suggested key words for referencing and acknowledgments, if any.

Manuscripts must be double-spaced and of letter-quality print. They must also use a type size of at least 12 characters per inch or 10 points. Please leave generous margins of at least 1 inch. All pages, including text, notes, and reference pages, must be numbered consecutively. All notes must be double-spaced and placed at the end of the manuscript as endnotes rather than footnotes.

Authors are responsible for securing permissions for all materials submitted. If more than 500 words of text are quoted from a book, or more than 250 words from an article, or if a table or figure has been previously published, the manuscript must be accompanied by written permission from the copyright owner.

Initial submissions of manuscripts may be sent by e-mail to *nhr@nursing. upenn.edu.* Contributors may also send 4 copies of their manuscripts via regular mail to the address below. Please send only clear copies of any photographs, tables, or figures at this point. All submissions will be acknowledged when received.

Final versions of manuscripts accepted for publication should be prepared in MS Word. The final packet submitted to the editorial offices of the *Review* must include: two hard copies of the final version and a version on disc; black-and-white, camera-ready glossy prints *or* TIF files with resolutions of at least 600 dpi of all photographs and figures; and all appropriate permissions and copyright releases.

All correspondence regarding manuscripts should be sent to: Patricia D'Antonio, RN, PhD, FAAN, Editor, *Nursing History Review,* University of Pennsylvania School of Nursing, 420 Guardian Drive, Room 307, Philadelphia, PA 19104-6096. Phone: 215/898-4502. Fax: 215/573-2168. E-mail: *dantonio@nursing.upenn.edu* or *nhr@nursing.upenn.edu.*

American Association for the History of Nursing, Inc.

Sandra Lewenson
President

Karen Egenes
First Vice President and
Chair, Strategic Planning
    Committee

Joy Buck
Second Vice President and
Chair, Program Committee

Barbara Gaines
Secretary

Laurie K. Glass
Treasurer

Susan Gunby
Director and
Chair, Publications Committee

M. Patricia Donahue
Director and
Chair, Awards Committee

Joan Lynaugh
Director and
Chair, By-Laws Committee

Brigid Lusk
Director and
Member, Finance Committee

Sylvia Rinker
Director, and
Member, Strategic Planning

Kathleen Hanson
Past President

Wanda C. Hiestand
Archivist

Janet L. Fickeissen
Executive Secretary

Requiem for *AJN*'s Place in the Profession

The American Nurses Association's (ANA) recent decision (March 2006) to sever its official ties with the *American Journal of Nursing (AJN)* saddened me. ANA's previous decision (1996) to sell *AJN* to the Lippincott Company (Lippincott Williams & Wilkins) for $24,000,000[1] horrified me. How much is a birthright worth?

There are moments in history when the paths of events, phenomena, and people intersect in such a way as to provide a focus of singular intensity and interest. The 1893 World's Fair in Chicago was such a moment for nursing. As chairman of the Hospital and Medical Section of the International Congress of Charities, Dr. John Shaw Billings appointed as chair of the nursing subsection his colleague at Johns Hopkins, Isabel A. Hampton, Superintendent of Nurses and Principal of the Training School for Nurses at Hopkins. In turn, Hampton carefully named the topics to be discussed, appointed the speakers, and arranged the programs for nursing's first professional meeting, and on a grand stage at that. [2] As Lavinia Dock, Hampton's assistant at Hopkins, described it later:

> In the programme [sic] of this section, of which the arrangement was to her a devoutly serious piece of work, may be found the seedlings of almost all the later lines of growth in the nursing profession in the United States. Nor was it accidentally so, but the result of most earnest thought and divination. Often as she planned to whom certain themes should be given, did she describe the whole possible future that might arise from the ideas she hoped to have brought out.[3]

Throughout the week, Hampton laid out her plans for the organization and advancement of nursing: "I hope that in the course of time we will be able to evolve Alumnae Associations, an American Nurses' Association, and a Superintendent's Convention. . ."[4] And so it occurred. The superintendents held their first meeting that very week, calling themselves the American Society of Superintendents of Training Schools (which, in 1952, became the National League for Nursing). The alumnae associations had numbered only six before the fair, but "once started, the founding of training school alumnae associations moved rapidly."[5] When the associations joined together in 1896 to form The Nurses Associated Alumnae of the United States and Canada (incorporated in 1911 as the ANA), Isabel Hampton Robb was elected the first president. Starting a graduate course for nursing instructors (at Teachers College in 1901) and founding a journal to communicate information and events (*The American Journal of Nursing* in 1900) followed in rapid order.

Five different journals for nurses had been published before 1901. The first, *The Nightingale*, 1886–1891, was edited by a Bellevue graduate who was also a physician. Starting in 1888, *The Trained Nurse and Hospital Review* (later renamed *The Nursing World*) appeared monthly for seventy years. Josephine Dolan, in *Nursing in Society*, described how, in 1889, it combined with the *Journal of Practical Nursing*, and later absorbed, one at a time, *The Nightingale, The Nurse, The Nursing World*, and *The Nursing Record*.[6]

But the *AJN* was the first journal managed entirely by nurses. Philip and Beatrice Kalisch told the story of the *AJN* in their history of American nursing. "In 1899," they wrote, "under the leadership of Mary E. P. Davis [and Sophia Palmer], a stock company was formed with about 550 cash subscriptions and a new journal, *The American Journal of Nursing*, . . . , made its debut in October 1900, and continues to the present."[7] America's first trained nurse, Linda Richards, purchased the first cash subscription.[8]

In 1912, the ANA purchased all the stock in order that the journal could be the official voice of the national nursing organization: "In order to secure freedom of expression of opinion or criticism, or advocacy of plan or policy in nursing matters, it became evident that the journal must be something more than an adjunct. It must be independent, unhampered by fear, favor or prejudice in its expressions of truths, as seen and interpreted by nurses. To that end it must be owned, edited, and controlled by nurses."[9] Some things should just never be for sale.

ELLEN D. BAER, RN, PhD, FAAN
Professor Emerita of Nursing
University of Pennsylvania
North Palm Beach, FL 33408

Notes

1. Diana Mason, RN, PhD, Editor of *AJN*, personal communication, April 24, 2006.
2. *Hospitals, Dispensaries and Nursing*, Papers and Discussions in the International Congress of Charities, Correction and Philanthropy, Section III, Chicago, June 12–17, 1893, Under the Auspices of the World's Congress Auxiliary of the World's Columbian

Exposition. John S. Billings, MD, and Henry M. Hurd, MD, eds. (Baltimore: The Johns Hopkins Press, 1894).

3. Lavinia L. Dock, *A History of Nursing,* Vol. III (New York: G.P. Putnam's Sons, 1912), 125–6.

4. Isabel A. Hampton et al., *Nursing of the Sick 1893* (New York: McGraw Hill, 1949), 157.

5. Arlowayne Swort, *The ANA: The Formative Years, 1875–1922,* unpublished doctoral dissertation (New York: Teachers College, 1973), 84–6.

6. Josephine A. Dolan, *Nursing in Society, A Historical Perspective,*   14 ed. (Philadelphia: WB Saunders, 1978), 272.

7. Philip A. Kalisch and Beatrice J. Kalisch, *The Advance of American Nursing* (Boston: Little Brown, 1978), 142–3.

8. Inaugural editor Sophia Palmer edited *AJN* until her death in 1920, when Mary M. Roberts assumed editorial direction. Nell V. Beeby followed Roberts in 1949 and oversaw the addition of two new journals, *Nursing Research* (1952) and *Nursing Outlook* (1953). Editors who followed Beeby included Jeannette White (1957), Edith Patton Lewis (1958–9), Barbara G. Schutt (1960–71), and Thelma M. Schorr (1971–81), who became president and publisher of AJNCo. (1981–90). By then, the company had added *Geriatric Nursing; MCN: The American Journal of Maternal Child Nursing; The International Nursing Index; the AJN Career Guide;* the *AJN Nursing Boards Review;* and the publications of the Educational Services Division to its standard.

9. Dolan, *Nursing in Society,* 272, quoting *The American Journal of Nursing and Its Company – A Chronicle, 1900–1975* (New York: American Journal of Nursing, 1975), 4.

Nursing History: Blurring Disciplinary Boundaries

When we examine the history of nursing, we take into consideration the broad components that affected its development: the labor market and labor laws, political issues of the day, the economy, religious and secular institutions and their influences on each other, gender relationships, and technological and scientific developments. We cannot just look at what happened, but rather we also need to explain how and why it occurred. At the same time, the complexities of health care and the knowledge explosion of the twenty-first century will bring new challenges to graduates of nursing and the health professions. This compels us as historians of nursing to develop, and to teach our students to develop, new ways of thinking about issues.

This article argues for a broad historical approach that takes an interdisciplinary view into consideration as we do our work in nursing history. Indeed, there is great potential for interdisciplinary study. Anne Marie Rafferty, Jane Robinson, and Ruth Elkan point out that nursing history "recognizes the inescapable social, political, economic, and cultural factors influencing nursing."[1] In this way, nursing history is linked to the social sciences and the humanities. It also has connections to anthropology, philosophy, literary criticism, ethnic studies, American studies, and women's studies.

In his book, *Historiography in the Twentieth Century: From Scientific Objectivity to the Postmodern Challenge*, Georg G. Iggers argues that the "concept of unified historical development on which a grand narrative" of history can be based, with its "confidence in progress," has broken down. Instead, historical narratives have found forms of expression that look more at power relationships, gender, culture, ethnicity, religion, and ideology. Invisible in the grand narrative are women's contributions, played out today in women's history, gender history, and feminist history.[2] These disciplines all have implications for nursing. For example, to understand why women compose the major nursing workforce and why so many immigrants found nursing attractive, it is important to study women's and immigration history. At the same time, historians of nursing can provide valuable insights for other disciplines regarding how women negotiated in a male-dominated health care system and created opportunities to expand their autonomy and the nursing profession over time.

Ethnic and immigration history can help us understand not only the lives of immigrant nurses but also the ways that different ethnic groups have been marginalized. This includes looking at the underlying links between immigration and public health. When historians study public health nursing, they can examine how society received immigrants in the past. Amidst the huge changes that immigration brought, nativist fears linked certain diseases to specific immigrants.[3] Did Irish, Filipino, Japanese, or other immigrant nurses to the United States face these social prejudices? Historians of immigration have variously described the immigrant experience. Did immigrant nurses go through an "uprootedness" and alienation, as Oscar Handlin portrayed early immigrant experiences?[4] Or a "transplantation," as John Bodnar described? To Bodnar and others, immigrants brought their own institutions that aided them in fashioning a life for themselves.[5] Finally, ethnic and immigration history help us understand changes in migrations and their global connections to the world.

Another area of scholarship includes oral histories about nurses' work. Women's history, anthropology, and sociology have also seen the collection of oral histories as important to their disciplines. Using strategies from cultural history that involve greater attention to language, Sherna Gluck and Daphne Patai, in *Women's Words: The Feminist Practice of Oral History*, assert that in analyzing the production of oral histories, the fields of speech communication and linguistics can be used. They also argue for using methods from contemporary literary theory that challenge "the older historian's tendency to see oral history as a transparent representation of experience." Rather, "the typical product of an interview is a text"; thus, "models of textual analysis" are needed.[6] Carried to an extreme, linguistic and textual analyses can deny reality altogether. To strict followers of this line of thinking, history loses its significance as human actors become irrelevant.[7] I am working from the assumption that we *can* learn something from our sources through careful scrutiny. At the same time, an examination of language can be used as a supplementary tool in nursing's oral history interpretations. Frequent uses of the statements, "We weren't allowed to. . .," "I didn't want to, but I had no choice," and "We had to do. . ." tells us about power relationships and the unwillingness of nurses to defy the authority figures in their daily life and work. However, the words, "I did it anyway" show their willingness to resist.[8] Through careful analysis of language, nurse historians can determine not only what nurses saw as important but also through what "ideological blueprints" they perceived their lives.[9]

Finally, when we teach nursing history, an interdisciplinary focus can serve as a guide for different interpretive lenses. French critic and philosopher Michel Foucault was concerned with institutions as producers of passive bodies.[10] Some historians of nursing have taken this interpretation to new levels as they examine nursing as a discipline of professionals who exercise power over society.[11]

This article briefly examines the implications of an interdisciplinary study of nursing history. Most important, in arguing for this broad perspective, it is important to note the common characteristics seen in contributions from different disciplines, revealing what Gluck and Patai call the "the artificiality of the academic division of knowledge."[12]

BARBRA MANN WALL, RN, PHD
Associate Professor of Nursing
University of Pennsylvania

1. Anne Marie Rafferty, Jane Robinson, and Ruth Elkan, *Nursing History and the Politics of Welfare* (New York: Routledge, 1997), p. i.

2. Georg G. Iggers, *Historiography in the Twentieth Century: From Scientific Objectivity to the Postmodern Challenge* (Middletown, CT: Wesleyan University Press, 1997), 57. He extends and critiques Peter Novick's *That Noble Dream: The "Objectivity Question" and the American Historical Profession* (Cambridge, UK: Cambridge University Press, 1993). See also Wendy K. Kolmar and Frances Bartkowski, *Feminist Theory: A Reader* (Boston: McGraw-Hill, 2005).

3. See, for example, Alan M. Kraut, *Silent Travelers: Germs, Genes, and the "Immigrant Menace"* (Baltimore: Johns Hopkins University Press, 1994); Nayan Shah, *Contagious Divides: Epidemics and Race in San Francisco's Chinatown* (Berkeley: University of California Press, 2001); John Harley Warner and Janet A. Tighe, *Major Problems in the History of American Medicine and Public Health* (Boston: Houghton Mifflin, 2001); and Jon Gjerde, *Major Problems in American and Immigration History* (Boston: Houghton Mifflin, 1998).

4. Oscar Handlin, *The Uprooted: The Epic Story of the Great Migrations That Made the American People* (New York: Little, Brown, and Co., 2002).

5. John Bodner, *Transplanted: A History of Immigrants in Urban America* (Bloomington: Indiana University Press, 1985). See also Warner and Tighe, *Major Problems,* 2. Other classical works in the history of immigration and ethnicity include Philip Gleason, *Speaking of Diversity: Language and Ethnicity in Twentieth-Century America* (Baltimore: Johns Hopkins University Press, 1992), and John Higham, *Strangers in the Land: Patterns of American Nativism,* 1860–1925 (New Brunswick, NJ: Rutgers University Press, 1994).

6. Sherna B. Gluck and Daphne Patai, *Women's Words: The Feminist Practice of Oral History* (New York: Routledge, 1991), 3. See also Elizabeth A. Clark, *History, Theory, and Text: Historians and the Linguistic Turn* (Cambridge, MA: Harvard University Press, 2004); and Barbra Mann Wall, "Textual Analysis as a Method for Historians of Nursing," *Nursing History Review, 14* (2006): 227–42.

7. Willie Thompson, *Postmodernism and History* (New York: Palgrave Macmillan, 2004); Peter Burke, *What Is Cultural History?* (Cambridge, UK: Polity Press, 2004); and Alan McKee, *Textual Analysis: A Beginner's Guide* (London: Sage, 2003).

8. Marie-Francoise Chanfrault-Duchet, "Narrative Structures, Social Models, and Symbolic Representation in the Life Story," in Sherna B. Gluck and Daphne Patai, eds., *Women's Words: The Feminist Practice of Oral History* (New York: Routledge, 1991), 77–99, especially 79.

9. Ibid., 90.

10. Michel Foucault, *The Birth of the Clinic: An Archeology of Medical Perception* (New York: Vintage Books, 1994); idem, *Madness and Civilization: A History of Insanity in the Age of Reason* (New York: Vintage Books, 1965); and idem, *Power/Knowledge: Selected Interviews & Other Writings 1972–1977,* ed. Colin Gordon (New York: Pantheon Books, 1980).

11. D. Gastaldo and D. Holmes, "Foucault and Nursing: A History of the Present," *Nursing Inquiry,* 6, no. 4 (1999): 231–40.

12. Gluck and Patai, *Women's Words,* 3.

From the Editor: In Appreciation to our External Reviewers

On behalf of the Editorial Review Board, I thank the following colleagues who gave generously of their time and expertise when asked to review manuscripts: Marita Bardenhager, Cynthia Connolly, Gerard Fealy, Linda Freeman, Christine Hallett, Kathleen Hanson, Brigid Lusk, Jane Schultz, Louise Selanders, and Susan Smith.

From Susan Benedict: Acknowledgements for "Maria Stromberger: A Nurse in the Resistance in Auschwitz," *Nursing History Review,* 14 (2006): 189–202.

I am indebted to Dr. Traute Page for accompanying me to the archives in Germany and Poland to obtain many of the documents used for this article. I thank both Dr. Page and Anette Hebebrand-Verner for their translation of archival documents. Drs. Thomas Wanger and Harald Walser, both of Austria, generously provided documents and advice. Without their research and publications, it is likely that Maria Stromberger's bravery would remain largely unknown. Dr. Wanger was the inspiration for the memory sign and wrote its inscription. Dr. Walser, along with Markus Barnay, was the producer of the television documentary about Maria Stromberger, "Engel von Auschwitz," that is cited in this article. I especially thank both Drs. Wanger and Walser for their assistance because this article would not have been possible without their generous help.

Rewriting Nursing History – Again?

CELIA DAVIES
King's College, London

In the late 1970s, when I first began to gather together the authors whose essays would later appear in *Rewriting Nursing History*,[1] I found myself among others who experienced the same kinds of dissatisfactions with the history of nursing that I did. With the arrogance of the young, we believed we were at the cutting edge, at the start of something new. The judgments of nurse historians have been kind; they seem to have confirmed us in the passions we displayed. Yet the themes, research designs, and methods that are in place today were simply not visible on the horizon. And perhaps it is quite right that that is so.

A critical reflection on what has transpired over the intervening years is an appropriate topic for this Monica Baly Memorial Lecture. At the time that I entered the world of nursing history in the United Kingdom, and for many years after that, Monica Baly was an indomitable figure. The wide-ranging arguments of her *Nursing and Social Change* were well known and stood alongside her standard text on district nursing, *An Approach to District Nursing*. There were what Sioban Nelson has called the "gentle corrections" to the existing canon in her book *Florence Nightingale and the Nursing Legacy* and a continuing array of articles and chapters came during the years thereafter.[2] It was Monica Baly who recorded the story of the re-emergence of nursing history of which *Rewriting Nursing History* was a part. Her careful documentation jolted my memory of those first visits I made to the Royal College of Nursing (RCN) library in London. It was there, with the assistance and encouragement of librarian Frances Walshe, that I began to put together the network of scholars that resulted in *Rewriting Nursing History*. But it was Baly who had the foresight and determination to put it all on paper and to work tirelessly behind the scenes with others such as Christopher Maggs to create an institutional presence for the history of nursing and to keep it alive.[3]

This article gives me an opportunity to reflect on the progress of nursing history since *Rewriting Nursing History* was published in 1980. There is no hope, in a context such as this, of doing justice to the impressive volume and range of work that has been accomplished over the years. What I will do, instead, is ponder some of the reflections of those who are steeped in the field. I will ask myself how far the approaches being advocated by them today relate to the demands of that youthful band who worked toward something I described as "more intellectually satisfying and at the same time more relevant to practising nurses too".[4] There are three parts to this article. First, I want to comment on the writing of *Rewriting Nursing History* and to trace how my own intellectual thinking about nursing – its past and its present – developed from and out of that. My training as a sociologist and student of social policy, rather than as an historian, is particularly germane to this. Second, I want to make some observations on a quarter-century of impressive achievements in the history of nursing. To help with that, I turn to four historiographic essays that have offered an overview at different points in the period raising issues – some of which differ and some of which remain the same. Third, I want to offer my own comments and observations on the current agenda – the themes and issues in the field and the circumstances under which nursing history is being produced.

An Intellectual Journey

Rewriting Nursing History was a book that fell into place not only as a result of conversations and correspondence with like-minded people in the worlds of academia but also with encouragement from the practicing nurses with whom I was in contact. We were in total agreement that it was time for a vibrant new kind of history, but we totally disagreed about the form that that history should take. My co-writers had strong commitments to labor history, Marxist history, and feminist history, to name a few. My concern at that time was not to advocate any one camp but to show that where you set up camp affected the view. I spent time attacking the conventional history that celebrated a path of advancement, pointing to it as a Whig version of history that needed to come into the open and face criticism and replacement. I challenged the coherent narrative accounts of seemingly uncontested and obvious facts. I argued that there was always a theory or at least a set of assumptions, and that it would be better for all of us if these came into the open. My authors agreed that it was important to help others see why we each started where we did and why we made our various methodological choices, hence opening up work to critique. My training had been as a sociologist with all the tendencies to reflection and relativism that that discipline brought. I admired the beautiful writing of those in the discipline of history, but I wanted to know where the methodology chapter was and what warrant there was – beyond elegance and coherence – for their accounts.

At the time, I had not set out to enter the field of nursing history, nor had I planned to edit a book. I had come, at the end of the 1960s, from a fascination with industrial sociology into research on hospital organization. The professional autonomy of doctors was to me the most visible feature of hospital life, and the concept of professions and the clash between profession and bureaucracy became the subject of my first published paper. However, nurses were also sociologically interesting. American nurses, placed by sociologists as a "semiprofession," seemed to be trying to take the route identified in the sociological work on professionalization, but British nurses were doing "the wrong thing" – going for a management hierarchy instead of seeking to gain control over education and the practice of their own work. I found the semiprofession concept unsatisfactory on several counts – so why not try to understand the historical trajectory of nursing in context in the two settings? I was confident that the secondary sources that I knew lined the shelves of the RCN library would allow me to fill the boxes of a neat comparative framework. The books disappointed, and the rest, of course, is history. That period saw a series of publications by me, making comparisons between United Kingdom and American nursing, struggling to make sense, for example, of the conceptual underpinnings of the categories of the United Kingdom census because I wanted to use its data, and going back to original sources to write on the challenges that faced Britain's General Nursing Council in the 1920s.[5]

I became a contract researcher, and my career took different directions. However, it was knowledge of the history of nursing that persuaded those in the United Kingdom Central Council for Nursing, Midwifery and Health Visiting (UKCC), the statutory body that maintains the professional register in the United Kingdom, that I was a fit candidate to work with them on the high-profile plan in the mid-1980s to try once again to reform nurse education in the United Kingdom. The historical understanding that I had developed of the directions of nurse education in Britain and the United States, as well as my command of a century of official and unofficial reports, gave me an edge, and I found myself for a period outside academe, with drafting responsibility for the report on the reform of nurse education, commonly known as "Project 2000".[6] This experience gave me an enduring sense of the importance of the long view that history can offer. But it also left me with a memory of the sense of frustration in the profession that nurses were just not being taken seriously. *Gender and the Professional Predicament in Nursing* was very much an outcome of this.[7] It is a book where my most obvious theoretical debts are to feminist theorists in diverse fields, including psychoanalysis and organization theory. My argument in a nutshell was that professionalization – in England, at any rate – was a nineteenth-century identity project of white, middle-class men that appealed to those who would not inherit land, giving them a sense of self-respect; that it was founded on a gender division; and that nursing is best understood as a gendered adjunct to a profession. As such, nursing was, and remained, in a deeply contradictory position as it tried to pursue a professional project of its own. This work was not history, but it had debts to historical scholarship as much as to feminist theory, which the chapters on education and on practice reveal most strongly. It could not have emerged without drawing on my historical understanding, but it also needed the feminist theory.

A more sustained piece of historical work came later with the invitation to produce a history of the UKCC and its contributions to the state regulation of nursing.[8] My colleague Abby Beach, who deserves much tribute for her part in that work, gave me an opportunity to see a trained historian at work and to log the dilemmas that an institutional history gives – with its inevitably messy archives and with the need to engage with those still deeply involved and tread the difficult path between celebration and critique. The sections between her "pure history" in Chapter One and my "policy relevance" in the final chapters were the product of much dialogue, where I constantly suggested lines of interpretation, and Abby, with her command over the sources, challenged them. Again, however, it has given me a stock of knowledge on which to reflect more as a sociologist and policy analyst than as a historian. My papers on regulation build out from this into a comparison with medicine, arguing against the equivalence of the two, underlining a significant difference between nurse regulation and medical regulation and seeing the legacies of the latter still tied with nineteenth-century gendered medical professional identity as contributing much to the present painful position of the General Medical Council in the United Kingdom.[9]

In sum, my excursions into history have been just that. I cannot claim full citizenship in the community of nursing historians. I have been more interested in the broadened perspective and the messages that might be carried out to nurses and to the policy world in which they find themselves today. I have also been concerned throughout with questions of subordination and oppression and the implications of this *both* for nurses *and* for the kind of health care available to us all. That shapes the agenda you hear about later in this article. But let me turn now to the achievements of the nursing history field.

Assessments of the Field – Different Times, Different Places

As an occasional sojourner in the history of nursing and a "late returner" to it in recent months, the transformation of the field since the early 1980s is amazing. There are full-length historical monographs on topics that were not even on the horizon as we began in the late 1970s to look at what was possible. There is methodological diversity and imaginative use of sources. There have been national and international conferences on the theme of the history of nursing; and the opportunities for networking that they offer have been grasped. Where there were no journals to consult in 1980, there are now several (although not all have managed to survive). Even a brief electronic search or two (a step unimaginable in 1980), to my pleasure and alarm, started to produce lists of very recent articles in double and triple figures. Nurses have managed to wrest time and training so the number of doctorates is growing. There has been an important, although small, continuation of interest among those trained as historians in the possibilities for understanding that are afforded by a study with a focus on nurses and nursing. Christopher Maggs was right to take me to task, seven years on, for worrying if there was enough for a follow-up book to *Rewriting Nursing History*.[10]

I want to agree with Patricia D'Antonio in her assessment that "understanding the work of nurses has reshaped historians' sense of the historical hospital, the treatment of disease, the birth of babies, and the role of women in their families and their communities".[11] It should have done so, and I suspect it will do so, but not yet. My judgment is more with Barbara Mortimer when she talks of the "scant attention" paid to nurses and their work and the rarity with which they figure in accounts to do with medicine and health.[12] To begin to engage with this growing corpus of work directly is a daunting task and not one to be undertaken lightly. Fortunately for me, something else that indicates the maturing of an intellectual discipline is the production of review essays that accomplish just that. I am going to focus briefly on four.

Janet Wilson James

Janet Wilson James, writing the essay, "Writing and Rewriting Nursing History" in 1984, provided the first of these.[13] I remember Janet and her partner, Ed, as the most hospitable and encouraging of people, with a wide network of academic friends and colleagues in the Boston area at that time; and she was one of the people who helped make possible the conference that led in 1983 to the collection *Nursing History: New Perspectives, New Possibilities*.[14] Her review paper sought to be a message carrier across into the world of medical history, citing these new publications and more besides. Nursing, said James, had had its past to itself, but life and thought were reviving. In that revival, she saw a place for different kinds of history and made a plea for nursing to engage with the mainstream and for the mainstream to engage with nursing. Later reviewers were differently positioned – all insiders to nursing, as well as contributors to the kind of scholarship and interchange that Janet James envisaged. If she had lived to see what followed, she would have been well satisfied.

Patricia D'Antonio

"Revisiting and Rethinking the Rewriting of Nursing History" by Patricia D'Antonio emerged in 1999.[15] (It was clear from this that these "re" word titles were going to get more challenging from here on in!) Sioban Nelson, in the third paper that I discuss, describes this publication as an "optimistic" account bringing us up to date with developments since the 1980s. Coming to it for the first time in preparing this lecture, however, I do not read it that way at all. It starts out optimistic with the comment about reshaping the thinking of historians that I have already cited. But it quickly goes on to be much more critical. For me, three points stand out. First, there was the comment that gender, class, and race were now there "however fleetingly" in nursing scholarship. "Yes!" I thought. Finding fleeting reference to gender has been the bane of my academic life. For me gender isn't fleeting, it makes a difference, a substantial difference to everything that follows. But she went on from there to talk of our comfort and complacency with what had become a paradigm of socially structured contradictions and passivity in the face of them. "Ouch!" I said to myself – she had authors such as Susan Reverby, Darlene Clark Hine, and Barbara Melosh in her sights[16] – she argued that we had not moved on – could this include me?

Her third point, and the one that was developed most fully throughout the essay, was that nursing "took on different meanings for different nurses at different times."[16a] We should acknowledge this by finding conceptual and analytical space to talk of identities that were not primarily driven by paid work. This line of argument was surely anathema to those who looked to and understood the lives of the elite leadership in nursing. But it was a wake-up call in terms of acknowledging the many, perhaps most, in nursing who wound their nursing work around lives connected to others – doing nursing, but not in a way that equated completely with entering and leaving the nexus of paid nursing work. "What," she said, "if we turn to issues raised in women's history and reposition identity rather than work at the center of our analysis of the relationships among nursing, gender and power?"[17] She was prompted in part by the scholarship of black feminists who had a different take on nursing from that of the white elite; she was also influenced by the work of Emily Abel. This was a name that led me to my bookshelves for a book I remembered as forging a path ahead of its time. *Circles of Care: Work and Identity in Women's Lives* was an interdisciplinary collaboration coming out of an American women's studies stable, feeling its way toward new ways of expressing lives of women untrammeled by the conceptual straightjacket of male careers.[18] D'Antonio's essay did indeed do much to bring the uninformed up to date with its citations of the scholarship between the mid-1980s and late 1990s. But it was more than that. It was deeply critical. Don't just study the leaders, do more and do better with your analysis of gender class and ethnicity. Remember that women have agency, too. I return to some of these themes later in the article.

Sioban Nelson

Sioban Nelson, like D'Antonio and unlike James, is positioned as an insider in the world of nursing. Her 2002 review paper, "The Fork in the Road: Nursing History Versus the History of Nursing," was a signal of the growing academic disciplinary times in that it appeared not in a medical history journal but in the *Nursing History Review*, an American journal at that point a decade old.[19] Nelson takes as her point of departure the overturning of the now familiar triumphalist account of nursing history and its replacement with cross-fertilization of ideas, from historians and from both modern and postmodern strands of theorizing in sociology. She asks what a decentered history would look like – that is, what would a history "minus its great women" look like? What happens if there is real acceptance of the proposition that all professions are self-serving? Nelson welcomes the diversity and plurality of nursing histories, and the injection of social theory. It is up to us, she says firmly to her peers, to "stop nursing from falling off the agenda of women's history and women's studies".[20] Her main points are several. First, she is keen not to dismiss the institutional histories, biographies, and organizational histories. This genre provides a vital record and resource for those who would do differently, and writings in this vein can also be treated as discursive activities – resources that serve to create meaning for their time through their narrative, sometimes consciously offering an identity to the novice nurse. Second, she insists that we do not reduce history to the use of a research technique or method of data collection: "Historical data," she argues, "are rendered meaningful only through the analysis of historical context. Historical sources are products of this historical context, and historical memory is fashioned by wider events, circumstances, and discourses".[21] In her sights are those who raid the past to bolster contemporary nursing theories. Argue with reference to the *historical* literature she orders and not the nursing science literature.

Nelson's nightmare is an increasing divide between enthusiastic nurses engaging in historical research from an ahistorical base and those who engage in disciplinary scholarship with little to say of interest to an audience beyond themselves. Underlying this – her third key point – is a question: who is nursing history for? Nelson's answer is that it must be for nurses, for the general public, and for historians themselves. As a new reader of this essay, I wonder about the impact her account of the Australian Nursing History Project, which she describes in some detail in the final section as seeking to make history relevant and accessible in schools and to a general public. Are there those who criticize its acknowledged "good old-fashioned professionalizing narrative"? Does the idea of multiple audiences and hence multiple kinds of history hold water?

Barbara Mortimer

Finally, I turn to an essay by Barbara Mortimer that serves as the introduction to *New Directions in the History of Nursing*, published in 2004.[22] Mortimer's wide-ranging scope and assessments of the field make it much more than a mere introduction. It is a review essay in itself, serving the dual function of challenging and reflecting in ways of interest to peers, while also being informative for newcomers. There are distinct echoes of the "who is it for?" question, but that aside, Mortimer is someone who wants more. The contribution that the history of nursing could make to the wider historiography of women is, she says, "yet to be fully realised" and the study of nurses in isolation "can seem like a defence mechanism".[23] "Looking beyond" is a phrase that recurs throughout the text. Criticism aside, she documents persuasively that the field is now both international and interdisciplinary, and that new approaches and methods are in play. That research questions deriving from historical and social science scholarship are now in use is amply confirmed by the range of contributions to the volume itself. But it is her agenda of topics and themes that is the focus of my concern.

In my reading of Mortimer's essay, two areas stand out: caring, and what she calls "the international agenda in relation to race and ethnicity." On caring, she notes growing calls to work on this "most important and most elusive topic." On internationalism and race and ethnicity, she argues that the struggle must be to relinquish the hold of Anglo-European thinking to yield a history from the point of view of the colonized. British work, she says, does not yet have the depth of that in the United States, but new work by differently positioned authors on colonial South Africa is highlighted, and her call for more work on the impact of in-migration to Britain in the 1950s is surely timely.[24] Mortimer has more on her agenda. On education and knowledge, I interpret her call as for a rebalancing – more on the history of knowledge than on the history of educational arrangements as such. On nursing and the military, she is looking for a path between glorifying the sacrificial heroine and a more "dispassionate eye." And what is her take on professionalization? There is reference to the complexity and the contradictions of a struggle for professional recognition and a depiction of this as an area where nursing has contributed to understanding gender (not a point, I suspect, that many feminist historians would choose to make). But is there something new and different to do? I am not sure.

A New Agenda?

These four essays by no means constitute the whole of the analytical commentaries on the field in a period of twenty-five years: the most cursory of glances at the *Nursing History Review* over the last few years shows how much debate is currently in play. There is both continuity and change, however, in the messages these essays convey. All want to mix with the mainstream, but they raise the questions: "Who is nursing history for?", "who should be doing it?", "does it need to change?", and "what about the hard messages to hear?" These are questions that need to fit in some way alongside the identification of both topics and theoretical frameworks.

I want to suggest a five-point agenda for the future, concerned both with some of the topics that the history of nursing is now engaged with and might engage with in the future and with some of the terms of that engagement – the struggles, intellectual and practical, that if not unique to this field are nonetheless ones with which those working in it need to hold nearer the forefront of their minds than hitherto.

My five areas are similar to the topics raised in *New Directions*,[25] but they are not quite identical, and what I want to say about them is perhaps more distinctive than the headings themselves. Both the topics and the commentary that I give are, of course, influenced by my own history and by my location in the United Kingdom, although these factors have a different weight for various topics. The contextualizing and perhaps discounting that readers do in light of this is at least as important as my remarks themselves.

The "Internationalism" of Nursing History

There are undoubtedly exciting developments afoot. In 1980, it was unimaginable that this field would have conferences that would attract international scholars, and that there would be journals featuring papers about nursing from countries around the globe and recognition of the considerable amount of boundary crossing by people and ideas in nursing. For me, this is a context in which the principal task is to rethink fundamental issues of subordination and oppression, and explore the way that inequalities of health and race, class, and gender work out, sometimes entirely unintentionally, as health care personnel and health care systems travel across an international stage. What stance should today's nursing historian have in regard to the themes of imperialism and colonialism, which are being revisited through theoretical work on postcolonial theory and globalization? Also, in what sense is it justified, if at all, to use today's theories to illuminate the past with its heady mix of ideologies of eugenics, racial superiority, and missionary zeal? Issues of race and ethnicity certainly must be to the fore here, but not to the exclusion of addressing the race/class/gender intersections in nursing and health care practice in contexts closer to home.

A different challenge of internationalization was best put for me in 1987 in Dublin by Irish feminist Ailbhe Smyth at the Third International Interdisciplinary Congress on Women. She said, and my half-remembered paraphrase cannot do justice to the elegance and the impact the original statement had, that she did not want our respectful silence and applause; instead, she wanted us to engage. But rarely it seems to me are we in a good position to engage. Conference attendees try to see similarities and differences, without enough background to do it well. They may do a real injustice to the thinking of a presenter struggling with a second language. We need to find some new practices if we are to generate real comparative understanding across national boundaries. I was intrigued to see an editorial in the journal *Gender and History* in 2002, emphasizing the value of publishing what it called the "jagged edges" – the debates and viewpoints of the real exchanges that conferences sometimes, but by no means always, facilitate. Does the polish that we all seek to apply to our papers in the end discourage the very debates we need to have? Perhaps "internationalism" deserves a conference to itself, reflecting nursing as the most traveled of women's professions and picking up directly on the multiple senses of internationalism and its potential.

Nursing, Health Policy, and the State

Over the years, nurses have repeatedly voiced complaints that they are not heeded in the world of health policy; reorganizations, innovations, and shifts in policy direction all seem to fail to acknowledge implications for nursing or to listen to a nursing voice. Recent years in the United Kingdom have seen a new development whereby nurses are invoked as a key resource to achieve government ends, as in nurse-led clinics and nurse prescribing. Often nurses are still uneasy, continue to believe their voices have not been heard, and conclude that they need "better leaders."

I believe there is considerable scope now for serious attention by nursing historians to the tracing of policy developments, perhaps making explicit comparisons of the contributions of doctors and nurses and attending to discourses that downgrade and devalue nurses and nursing. Such work may well cause us to rethink some of those standard accounts of health policy development. An upcoming history of the RCN will reveal more than we know already about some of the lobbying activity by nurses.[26] But, to my knowledge, no one is looking at the potential for exploring official records on key twentieth-century policy debates for what these might reveal about the positioning of nursing and visions of what kind of health care is needed. I am thinking here of the absence of overt debate about nursing in the formation of the National Health Service and in the reports on its functioning and its successive reorganizations, as well as perhaps of how the profession figures in developments in particular policy fields – mental health, care of the elderly, and so on. The government archive, the memoirs of ministers and civil servants, and official reports and transcripts of parliamentary debates remain to be mined for what they say about prevailing attitudes and the issues with which the profession has had to contend.[27]

To do this well requires an understanding of political ideologies and parties, central and local government relations, and how nursing, health policy, and the state intersect in their concerns. I am reminded of Michael Moran's comparative work on Britain, Germany, and the United States,[28] where he argues that health care systems always pose problems for the state and urges us to see the state and professions not as locked in a power battle but as "wound round each other" and mutually constituting each other. His focus, of course, is on medicine, but I suspect there is another part of the story, a different winding around of both state and medicine, that involves nursing and that enables medicine and the state to relate to each other in the way that they do. One key point that he makes is that there are, of course, different understandings of the role of the state and its institutions and structures between different countries. Sociologists tell me there is the Anglo-American concept of professions versus the continental one – I have yet to see this fleshed out effectively in relation to the health care professions.

Not Professionalization But Professional Identity?

I am not sure that professionalization, as some inexorable process followed by one occupational group after another, is a concept that deserves to detain us much longer. Changing notions of professional identity, what it means when someone says they are a doctor, a nurse, a lawyer, an architect, and so on, however, are a different matter. I am on record (as noted previously) as arguing that what it was to be a middle- and upper-class man in the nineteenth century and what it was to be a doctor were deeply intertwined. Medical men's sense of self-respect at that time involved their place at the head of the household, together with mastery of scientific knowledge and a positioning of the work of the nurse as handmaid. I have been struck by how, in a mid-twentieth-century public inquiry into the regulation of the medical profession, the emphasis on preserving the self-respect of the profession was still being articulated and, indeed, was clearly shared among the scientists, lawyers, and doctors present.[29]

If we could find ways of gaining more access to notions of self and identity within the medical profession, through diaries and correspondence perhaps, we would understand better what it was that the early nurse professionalizers faced. Historians have documented overt antiwomen sentiment, but they have said little from the angle that such sentiment is simultaneously constitutive of masculinity. New work needs to attend to theoretical developments in the study of identity and identities. Such work would mean working toward an understanding of doctoring and nursing as deeply interrelated – I have long tried to argue that one cannot be adequately understood without the other. Furthermore, the way in which identity is constructed through binary thought, through devaluing an "other," needs to be faced more directly.[30] Identities research, furthermore, is an important locale where attention to ethnicity, class, and race is currently occurring.

Nursing Practice, Nursing Knowledge, and Caring

In nursing history to date, interest in the politics of nursing had far outweighed interest in its practice. If I ask myself what the circumstances of nursing practice have been at different times – my answer has to be "severely circumscribed." The dominance of medicine, student labor systems in hospitals, and the high rate of trained to untrained are among the features I identified when I argued in *Gender and the Professional Predicament* that nurses in the United Kingdom, until recently, faced the "polo mint problem" – once trained, they spend time supervising others more than practicing nursing. For me, any history of changing practice must be seen in this light. Working to doctors' orders, with an education base entangled with service, nurses have run the risk of denying their own agency, but commentators on nursing also risk falling into the converse traps of overcelebrating or overblaming nurses.

Where does this take me? There is talk of potential work on the history of nursing research. Perhaps this is an area where nursing historians might engage with medicine and with the division of labor in medical research where nurses appear as data gatherers and research assistants whose contributions are too easily overlooked in stories of clever clinicians and pioneering scientists. Is there a DNA story, a Rosalind Franklin story, to be told?[31] Other kinds of collaborative work on the boundaries between nurses and allied health professions perhaps fit somewhere here. The history of physiotherapy techniques and of the knowledge base of dietetics, both intertwined with practicalities of hospital care and its changing division of labor, are topics that might be examined under the practice head.

When addressing the practicalities and realities of doing nursing, the topic of the ratios of trained and untrained nurses, as well as the battle in nursing to replace the latter with the former, needs to come into stronger focus. It is high time, in my view, for nurse historians to take a critical look at what has happened throughout the years to those who have worked both as nurses with less than a full registration training and in roles nominally, at least, as assistant to the nurse. I recently invited Carole Thornley, author of a series of research projects on care assistants for Union, the British trade union, to bring together this work for a collection of essays on the future health care worker. The comments that her survey respondents made were heart-rending – not only for the juggling that they did to live on minimal pay but also for the absence of recognition of the bedside nursing that they were undertaking and for their hunger to learn more about this.[32] Trying to improve its position, nursing has been "between a rock and a hard place",[33] but when care assistants report that they have taken nursing textbooks home to try to teach themselves about the patients for whom they are caring, something has gone very wrong. They deserve at least a "history from below" that acknowledges this and that also, in the United Kingdom setting, addresses the treatment of enrolled nurses as second class, a story that we know was compounded in the 1950s by the exploitation of recruits who came by invitation from the West Indies to the United Kingdom.

Writing on the practice of nursing, referring to the work of Reverby and to an agenda-creating essay by Maggs, Mortimer calls for direct attention to care and caring as a topic.[34] In my remarks in this article, I have sought to find another path. Reverby's argument that nurses have been "ordered to care in a society that does not value caring" was a tremendously powerful insight at the time and remains so. But to move us on, focusing on the realities of nursing knowledge and practice and the specificities of how these have and have not been constrained, I suspect, may offer a better route now for understanding a group that remains subordinated in the division of labor and itself often subordinates others.

Living Lives as Nurses

This is a theme that D'Antonio introduced in her 1999 essay and has pursued further in her recent research. She invites us to consider lives as lived by nurses – lives, that is, lived in their totality, and not lives lived solely as nurses doing the paid work of nursing. This is a theme that brings attention to the full diversity of those who do nursing and asks what nursing means for them, their relatives and friends, and the communities in which they live. It is a theme that cries out for biographical and autobiographical work, urging historians of nursing to engage with today's strong currents of work in oral history and the complexity of narrative accounts. It is a theme that asks us to think about potential sources in new ways. What letters and diaries are there for twentieth-century nurses that we have still to find and exploit? This is also a theme that brings the corpus of theoretical work on identities – which I mentioned earlier – firmly into frame. Furthermore, it certainly has a capacity to illuminate the present – what today policy makers call the work-life balance – a concept that has only come into use in recent years, and which, if used with care, might shed more light on the past.

Whatever the topics in which the history of nursing engages in the coming years, there will be cross-cutting challenges that continue to need to be addressed. First, nursing's invisibility to policy makers and to academics means that historians need to take an oppositional stance and to be working against the grain, not just adding but reconceptualizing. Second, to achieve this, they will need to look out for theoretical work from gender studies, black studies, postcolonial thinking, or wherever that has the capacity to illuminate this. To work from and with a position of subordination and oppression is to be an academic boundary crosser and convention breaker. Third, I see nurse historians and historians of nursing as not only carrying out historical scholarship but also still, to an important extent, fighting to establish the conditions under which that scholarship is possible. In short, they will need to be both skeptical of abstract theory and committed to engaging with it; and they will need to be writing for multiple audiences – for historians, nurses, and a wider public that reads history.

Conclusion

I titled this article "Rewriting Nursing History – Again?" because each new generation must engage in rewriting history, and the rewritings that we produce will be affected by our own identities, our subject positions, and the discourses of the day. Yes, we do see things differently from those who came before us. We earnestly think that we see further, more, and better (as I and my coauthors did in 1980). But then others come along to put us in a social and intellectual context that we ourselves were unable to see.

I cannot end without a reference once again to Monica Baly. I do not know whether she would have approved of what I have had to say. In fact, she might have seen me as altogether too sociological for her taste. She might have admonished us – less reflection and more activity. I suspect, however, that she would have been an avid listener to all the conference papers. And more than once, she would have been the first to jump up, comment, and challenge. She was an enlivening presence. She is sorely missed.

CELIA DAVIES, BA, MA, PhD
Visiting Professor
Nursing Research Unit
King's College, London

Acknowledgments

This article is a revised version of the Monica Baly Lecture, given at the conference "Nursing History: Profession and Practice" held at the University of Manchester, November 18, 2005, and organized by the United Kingdom Centre for the History of Nursing and Midwifery, University of Manchester, and by the History of Nursing Society of the Royal College of Nursing. I want to thank the organizers for suggesting the idea of reflecting on twenty-five years of development since the publication *Rewriting Nursing History*. I am particularly grateful to Patricia D'Antonio for her enthusiasm, effort, and encouragement in the process of revising the manuscript for publication.

Notes

1. Celia Davies, ed., *Rewriting Nursing History* (London: Croom Helm, 1980).
2. Three major texts by Monica Baly, each running to multiple editions, are *Nursing and Social Change* (London: Heinemann Medical, 1973); *An Approach to District Nursing* (London: Heinemann Medical, 1981); and *Florence Nightingale and the Nursing Legacy* (London: Croom Helm, 1986). She published on a wide range of more specific historical topics, including hospital nursing, district nursing in the Queen's Nursing Institute, and the impact of the Nightingale Fund on nurse education, and she provided biographical sketches of a number of key individuals.
3. See Monica Baly, "A Brief History of the RCN History of Nursing Society and Its Journal, 1983–1994. Part One. The Early Years," *History of Nursing Society Journal*, 1, no. 2 (1995):75–82. This journal was superseded by the *International History of Nursing Journal* in 1995, under the editorship of Christopher Maggs. Sadly, this journal came to an end after seven volumes as a result, the then-editor explained, of the economic climate, library finances, and of not being seen as central to nursing education. For more on Monica Baly, see Christopher J. Maggs, "Reflections in the Life of Monica Baly," *International History of Nursing Journal*, 4, no. 2 (1998–9): 41–5.
4. Davies, *Rewriting*, 9.
5. These publications appeared in a diversity; of places. Some were deliberately addressed to a policy and practice audience in nursing; see, for example, "Continuities in the Development of Hospital Nursing," *Journal of Advanced Nursing*, 2 (1977): 479–93; "Four Key Events in Nursing History," *Nursing Times*, 74 (1978): 65–72. Other publications appeared in more conventional discipline-related publications related both to history and to social science; see, for example, "Making Sense of the Census in Britain and the USA: The Changing Occupational Classification and the Position of Nurses," *Sociological Review*, 18 (1980): 581–609; "The Regulation of Nursing Work: An Historical Comparison of Britain and the USA," in J. Roth, ed., *Research in the Sociology of Health Care, Volume 2: Changing Structures of Health Service Occupations* (Greenwich, CT: JAI Press, 1982); "Professionalizing Strategies as Time- and Culture-Bound: American and British Nursing, Circa 1893," in Ellen Condliffe Lagemann, ed., *Nursing History: New Perspectives, New Possibilities* (New

York: Teachers College Press, 1983); "The Health Visitor as Mother's Friend: A Woman's Place in Public Health, 1900–1914," *Social History of Medicine*, 1 (1988): 38–57.

6. For areas where this work drew especially on historical perspectives, see "UKCC Project 2000, Educational Policy Advisory Committee," in *United Kingdom Central Council for Nursing, Midwifery and Health Visiting (UKCC) Project 2000: A New Preparation for Practice* (London: The Council, 1986); "The Enrolled Nurse: Looking Back and Looking Forward," *Project Paper 4* (London: The Council, September 1984). For a comment on the extent to which the project lent itself to the generation of historical records, see "Project 2000 – A Word to Tomorrow's Historian," *History of Nursing Bulletin*, 2 (1988): 2–8.

7. Celia Davies, *Gender and the Professional Predicament in Nursing* (Buckingham: Open University Press, 1995).

8. Celia Davies and Abigail Beach, *Interpreting Professional Self-Regulation: A History of the UKCC* (London: Routledge, 2000).

9. See, for example, "What About the Girl Next Door? Gender and the Politics of Professional Self-Regulation," In G. Bendelow, M. Carpenter, C. Vautier, and S.J. Williams, eds., *Gender, Health and Healing* (London: Routledge, 2002); "Registering a Difference: Changes in the Regulation of Nursing," In J. Allsop and M. Saks, eds., *Regulating the Health Professions* (London: Sage, 2003).

10. Christopher Maggs, ed. *Nursing History: The State of the Art* (London: Croom Helm, 1987).

11. Patricia D'Antonio, "Revisiting and Rethinking the Rewriting of Nursing History," *Bulletin of the History of Medicine*, 73 (1999): 269.

12. Barbara Mortimer, "Introduction. The History of Nursing: Yesterday, Today and Tomorrow," in Susan McGann and Barbara Mortimer, eds. *New Directions in the History of Nursing* (London: Routledge, 2004): 1.

13. Janet Wilson James, "Writing and Rewriting Nursing History," *Bulletin of the History of Medicine*, 58 (1984): 568–84.

14. Ellen Condliffe Lagemann, ed. *Nursing History: New Perspectives, New Possibilities* (New York: Teachers College Press, 1983). The volume arose from papers presented at a conference hosted by the Rockefeller Archive Centre.

15. D'Antonio, "Revisiting and Rethinking," 268–290.

16. Barbara Melosh, *The Physician's Hand: Work, Culture and Conflict in American Nursing* (Philadelphia: Temple University Press, 1982); Susan M. Reverby, *Ordered to Care: The Dilemma of American Nursing, 1850–1945* (New York: Cambridge University Press, 1987); Darlene Clark Hine, *Black Women in White: Racial Conflict and Cooperation in the Nursing Profession* (Bloomington: Indiana University Press, 1989).

16. D'Antonio, "Revisiting and Rethinking," 272.

17. D'Antonio, "Revisiting and Rethinking," 279.

18. Emily K. Abel and Margaret K. Nelson, eds. *Circles of Care: Work and Identity in Women's Lives* (Albany: The State University of New York Press, 1990).

19. Sioban Nelson, "The Fork in the Road: Nursing History Versus the History of Nursing," *Nursing History Review*, 10 (2002): 175–88.

20. Nelson, "Fork," 185.

21. Nelson, "Fork," 181.

22. Mortimer, "Introduction," 4–5.

23. Mortimer, "Introduction," 5, 7.

24. Mortimer, "Introduction," 9.

25. Mortimer and McGann's *New Directions* begins with the essay by Mortimer under discussion and ends with a chapter by Joan E. Lynaugh in "Common Working Ground," which suggests eight topics for the future, adding "things to worry about."

26. This work is currently in preparation, Susan McGann, Rona Dougall, and Anne Crowther, and is tentatively titled, *Creating an Identity for Nurses: A History of the Royal College of Nursing* 1916–1989.

27. For a contemporary critical analysis of official policy on nursing policy, see Celia Davies, "Political Leadership and the Politics of Nursing," *Journal of Nursing Management*, 12, no. 4 (2004): 235–41. For insights into the power of in-depth discourse analysis, see M. Wetherell, S. Taylor, and S.J. Yates, eds., *Discourse Theory and Practice* (London: Sage, 2001); M. Wetherell, S. Taylor, and S.J. Yates, eds., *Discourse as Data* (London: Sage, 2001). For some early suggestive comments on the revealing and "unflattering" nature of civil servant memoranda when discussing nursing, see Davies and Beach, "Interpreting," 19, note 8.

28. Michael Moran, *Governing the Health Care State: A Comparative Study of the UK, the US and Germany* (Manchester, UK: Manchester University Press, 1999).

29. Report of the Committee of Inquiry into the Regulation of the Medical Profession, Cmnd. 6018, HMSO, 1975 (Merrison Report).

30. For a classic collection of theoretical essays, see Stuart Hall and Paul Du Gay, eds., *Questions of Cultural Identity* (London: Sage, 1995). An analysis seeking to demonstrate contemporary relevance for health practitioners can be found in Celia Davies, "Workers, Professions and Identities," in J. Henderson and D. Atkinson, eds., *Managing Care in Context* (London: Routledge, 2003).

31. For some accounts of the place of Rosalind Franklin in the story of the discovery of DNA and the hurdles that were put in her way, see, for example, B. Maddox, *Rosalind Franklin: The Dark Lady of DNA* (New York: Harper Collins, 2002); and Lynne Osman Elkin, "Rosalind Franklin and the Double Helix," *Physics Today*, 56 (2003): 42–8.

32. Carole Thornley, "What Future for Health Care Assistants: High Road or Low Road?" in Celia Davies, ed., *The Future Health Workforce* (London: Palgrave, 2003).

33. See Nona Y. Gazer, "Between a Rock and a Hard Place": Women's Professional Organizations in Nursing and Class, Racial, and Ethnic Inequalities," *Gender and Society*, 5, no. 3 (1991): 351–71.

34. See Mortimer, "Introduction," 9–10; Reverby, "Ordered to Care"; Maggs, "A History of Nursing: A History of Caring," *Journal of Advanced Nursing*, 23 (1996): 630–5.

ARTICLES

Florence Nightingale's Nursing Practice

Joyce Schroeder MacQueen
Laurentian University

Why is the woman who is credited as the founder of modern nursing considered by many scholars not to have actually nursed after her return from the Crimea? This article examines the ways Florence Nightingale's nursing has been deprecated or ignored in the literature and tries to redress this failure by uncovering Nightingale's nursing practice in the 1870s, 1880s, and into the 1890s. I examine her nursing as provided to Holloway villagers, cottagers on the Lea Hurst property, employees at Lea Hurst and Claydon, and members of her extended family. I also argue that her concern for the health of the Lea Hurst/Holloway people and her beliefs about nursing caused her to initiate reform of nursing at the Buxton Hospital, where her patients were admitted. The situation in Buxton in 1878 and 1879 provides an interesting example of Nightingale's reform *modus operandi*.

Florence Nightingale was born in Florence, Italy, on May 12, 1820, while her parents were on an extended honeymoon. Her sister, Parthenope, had been born in Naples a year earlier. Obviously, her parents, Frances and William Edward Nightingale (known in the literature as Fanny and W.E.N.), were wealthy. When the Nightingales returned to England, they settled in Derbyshire on the beautiful property W.E.N. had inherited outside Holloway village. Compared to estates such as nearby Chatsworth, Lea Hurst was modest, and so it eventually became only their summer home. The rest of the year they lived in the much grander Embley Park in Hampshire or in London during the appropriate season. Lea Hurst, however, was Florence Nightingale's favorite, and she developed relationships with the estate's cottagers and villagers that continued throughout her life.

Nightingale was educated by her father, who had studied at Cambridge. She was fluent in seven languages and had a bent for mathematics and statistics. Very

Nursing History Review 15 (2007): 29–49. A publication of the American Association for the History of Nursing. Copyright © 2007 Springer Publishing Company.

early in her life, she realized she could not abide the boredom of the role accorded to wealthy women. As she struggled with finding her own place in life, she came to feel that God was calling her to a career in nursing. Nightingale was thirty-one before her family reluctantly assented to her training to be a nurse because British nurses were seen as unsavory and British hospitals as unfit for ladies. In 1851, she went to Germany to the deaconess institute in Kaiserswerth, where she trained for three months. She worked for a year as head of the Institute for the Care of Sick Gentlewomen on Harley Street in London. In keeping with nineteenth-century practice for middle-class women, Nightingale was never remunerated for her work.

Then came the Crimean War of 1854–56 and Nightingale's claim to fame. Her nursing of the soldiers in the war made her a legend before she arrived back in England, exhausted from the incessant work and debilitated from the aftermath of a fever. She was, in varying degrees, unwell for the rest of her life. All her work was carried out within and despite the limitations of her physical condition. The Crimean War was a pivotal point in her life. It set her on the world stage and gave her long-term meaningful work. She worked at reforming the military medical system and its education. The Nightingale Fund, established to honor her work in the Crimea, provided the means and stimulus to develop a program for training nurses. In addition, she worked on sanitation in India, hospital statistical records, public health, and community nursing. These projects resonated worldwide and still command the limelight in the Nightingale literature, but they have overshadowed the more private sphere of action with the villagers around Lea Hurst and with her family.

Nightingale's nursing is often overlooked, not only because of the smaller private sphere of action but also because many researchers consider her work as a nurse insignificant. F.B. Smith, for example, dismisses her nursing of the cottagers around Lea Hurst as "her impulsive ventures into local village nursing," despite the extensive correspondence with Dr. C.B.N. Dunn over a period of some twenty years.[1] Sue M. Goldie also uses the term "impulsive" as a blanket description of Nightingale's nature but credits her with being a "born reformer."[2] Martha Vicinus and Bea Nergaard downplay any of Nightingale's nursing after Kaiserswerth and perhaps some work in the Crimea. They subscribe to the myth that Nightingale never left her bed after Crimea, despite readily available knowledge that she traveled regularly to Embley Park, the family home in Hampshire, to Lea Hurst in Derbyshire, and to Claydon House in Buckinghamshire. At Embley, in fact, Nightingale gave physical care to her dying mother. Vicinus and Nergaard conclude that, because Nightingale worked through letters and interviews, she was isolated from current events and obsolete.[3] Overall, in fact, they seem to limit nursing to hands-on activity and ignore the broader definition to which Nightingale subscribed.

Nightingale on Nursing

Writing from Crimea in 1856, Nightingale described the nursing she was attempting to make possible. She explained that she had settled with the doctors so the nurses in Balaclava "should be allowed to do the needful for the sick, give all the extras (and cook them), all the medicines and the wine and brandy and see to the cleanliness of the patients. These four things, the extras, medicines, stimulants and cleanliness were the chief points."[4] Nightingale was negotiating with the doctors, managing the nurses who were carrying out these functions, and also procuring many of the supplies that were used.

In 1859, in her *Notes on Nursing*, she expands on her definition of nursing. This book was written not for nurses but for "women who have personal charge of the health of others." Here, Nightingale dealt with providing a health environment (chapter headings are ventilation, warming, cleanliness, noise, light, beds and bedding, and variety), personal cleanliness, and food. Nightingale referred to all this as "*sanitary* nursing," not the "handicraft" of nursing, which dealt with skills such as dressings and medicines. Both sanitary and handicraft nursing were necessary for nurses. Nightingale commented, "A patient may be left to bleed to death in a sanitary palace."[5] In addition, Nightingale stressed the importance of management, what she referred to as "Petty Management." By this, she meant assuring "that what you do when you are there, shall be done when you are not there."[6] It was not the devoted nurse working extra hours that would produce the best care but the nurse who had the art of "multiplying herself" to ensure good care when she was not there.

Nightingale's broad view of nursing is evident in her appraisal of nursing in Kaiserswerth, where she trained in 1851. Later in life, she claimed that the nursing there was "nil," although her clinical notes show that patients were, in fact, nursed.[7] What Kaiserswerth did not have was a *system* of nursing. Nurses reported to religious authorities, not to nurses. Decisions were based on religion, not on nursing principles or medicine.[8] Nightingale's idea of the importance of the total system became part of her approach to nursing reform. Nurses from her program at St. Thomas' Hospital were never sent out alone to another institution. Always a group with a superintendent or head nurse was sent out. It was the system that required improvement, not just the nursing of individual patients.[9]

Nightingale was not alone in defining nursing broadly. Sir Henry Wentworth Acland, Regius Professor of Medicine at Oxford, in the introduction to Florence S. Lees' *Handbook for Hospital Sisters*, wrote, "Nursing consists of (1) cleaning (patients, beds, furniture etc.) 'housemaid's work,' (2) tending sick patients, dressings, posture, medicines, tempers to be soothed, carrying out orders of physicians and surgeons, (3) work of one organizing mind to superintend and regulate the steady harmonious action of one or of several such wards – to sum up superintendence, ministration and housework."[10] In late nineteenth-century America, too, the idea of nursing was seen largely as management. Tom Olson and Eileen Walsh, in their examination of the nature of nursing in an American nursing program in 1892 to 1937, found that "handling the sick, managing other workers, and controlling the ward, all to produce neat, finished-appearing work, were responsibilities that held consistent to the nurses' frequently stated ideals of physical and mental stamina and skill."[11]

Gillian Gill, along with F.B. Smith, describes Nightingale as "dreaming of power" from an early age, claiming that "By the early 1840s, power was already a key concept for Florence Nightingale."[12] Nursing neighbors might give an unoccupied woman a sense of power, but it would not do that for a woman on the world stage as Nightingale was. Smith and Gill, therefore, attempting to show Nightingale's craving for power, are bound to ignore her low-key work with neighbors. Gill, however, credits Nightingale with having "all the makings of a great clinician," being adept, for example, at applying leeches even before she went to Kaiserswerth.[13] Even Barbara Montgomery Dossey, who is sympathetic to Nightingale's nursing, ignores the work with villagers and the Buxton Hospital. She does, however, identify Nightingale's "gift for large-scale systems analysis" as the basis for her reforms.[14]

Possibly another reason for ignoring Nightingale's nursing of villagers and family is that the archival sources are scattered. The Dunn correspondence is located primarily at the Derbyshire Record Office in Matlock, not far from Lea Hurst and Buxton. The Verney Papers, which are rife with descriptions of Nightingale's care of ill relatives, are at Sir Harry Verney's home, Claydon House. Sir Harry was Parthenope's husband and was a widower with grown children when they were married. Florence Nightingale had her own room with a bell for summoning servants at Claydon. Sir Harry was a member of the Nightingale Fund Committee and for many years its chair, and Nightingale corresponded regularly. Claydon is, therefore, a significant source of data on Nightingale's nursing of her family. Claydon is now a National Trust property and, although not far from London, is in the country without available public transportation. The archive is only open the first Monday of the month by appointment.

Some of the sources are more readily at hand; for example, the Wellcome Institute for the History of Medicine, the London Metropolitan Archives, and the British Library are in London. Copies of some of the Claydon materials are available at the Wellcome Institute. But even London entails expensive travel for the North American researcher. Fortunately, The Collected Works of Florence Nightingale Project will soon have these materials available electronically. This will widen the possibility of research into barely tapped aspects of Nightingale's life.[15] All these archival sources were consulted for this article.

Nightingale and Nursing

It was usual in the nineteenth century for the wealthy to be concerned about the welfare of the poor living in their neighborhoods, whether tenants on their property or nearby villagers. Without social safety networks, illness and un-employment made such philanthropy essential. Gertrude Himmelfarb, writing of Victorian philanthropists, states that they were "personally involved in the day-to-day lives of the poor," and that "they brought to their work a spirit of professionalism."[16]

As a child, Florence Nightingale learned this concern by visiting poor people with her father, her mother, or Aunt Julia, her mother's sister. In fact, Aunt Julia "kept track" of the illnesses and specific needs of families.[17] As a teenager, Nightingale visited the poor herself, but in the 1870s and 1880s, when she was living in London and only occasionally at Lea Hurst, she had a network of informants to keep her in touch with these neighbors. Through Mr. Yeomans, the Lea Hurst estate manager, she provided a roster of neighbors with meat, milk, and nourishments such as "cocoatine" (a nourishing drink) and broth. Sometimes she provided material for them to sew their own clothes. She established a plan to assist the young working girls to save money by matching their savings with her own money. She and Dr. Dunn established a coffeehouse to keep the men from spending their money on alcohol. These activities were all part of her obligation as a wealthy woman, what is commonly referred to as noblesse oblige. Because Nightingale was a nurse, however, she went beyond this kind of benevolence and nursed those who were ill. That is, in the broad sense of nursing, she managed their care.

Some of her letters give an indication of the amount of time and money she spent on these nursing activities. In 1879, in a letter to Fred Verney, Sir Harry's son, she stated, "Lea Hurst costs me £500 a year, chiefly among the old & sick women: (the Doctor's Bill alone is £160 a year)."[18] In 1881, she wrote, "I have

16 more afternoons I must give to the village people here—then rest a day or two—then come to London."[19] Clearly, when she was at Lea Hurst and well enough, she visited the villagers personally. Most of the year, however, she nursed by mail. Nightingale had a number of correspondents who kept her in touch with the condition of her patients. She used the information mailed or reported to her and, with her knowledge of the patients and the diseases and infirmities they presented, decided on the kind of care needed. Then she consulted with Dr. Dunn about the care required.

In writing to Dunn, Nightingale often referred to an individual patient as "your patient," but, when she referred to the whole group, she called them "our patients."[20] Although Dunn was on site, she informed him in her letters of the condition of the patients, the progress or not that they were making, and possibilities of treatment. Even when she was at Lea Hurst and Dunn came for lunch, she nevertheless asked him for a written report on the patients. She requested him to make home visits and paid him quarterly for his services. She saw her work with Dunn as a partnership. There are more than ninety Nightingale letters to Dunn, mostly written in the 1870s and 1880s. They were usually two or three pages in length, but sometimes they were much longer and present a picture of a warm relationship between the two. The letters provided progress notes on all the patients at that time and showed a depth of caring about the overall lives of the villagers. Nightingale understood the effect of illness and infirmity on activities of daily living, on family relationships, and on family finances. The brief excerpts given here give some of the flavor of these relationships.

In October 1876, when Nightingale was at Lea Hurst, she wrote to Dunn at 6 A.M. to report that Mrs. Swindell, a typhoid patient, had swollen ankles and feet and was planning to go to her sister's home. A week later, she asked Dunn to visit Mrs. Swindell, who was still in her own home, and also Widow Henstock, "who is said to have vomited blood a few days ago."[21] In the same letter, she invited Dunn for luncheon and asked for a written report on Mrs. Swindell, Widow Henstock, and the girl Holmes.

The next summer, when Nightingale was back at Lea Hurst, she informed Dunn by letter, "I understand that Adelaide Peach, the girl with Pericarditis, has bed sores. If this be so, you probably know it. Would you wish her to be put on a Water-bed or water-pillow: and if so where could either be had?"[22] Dunn obviously visited immediately because the next day Nightingale wrote him asking where to get the powders he had ordered for the bed sore and where to get a water pillow if he were to order it.[23] The next year, Nightingale requested Dunn "to call upon the sister of Adelaide Peach – who died last year: I am told she is very ill."[24]

Later that same August, Nightingale asked Dunn to visit Mrs. Broomhead, a woman with an "incurable goiter" who was in severe pain.[25] In October 1878, she wrote, "should you think it possible that Widow Broomhead might undergo an operation in London? If not, how long is she likely to live, & what, poor woman, will be her end?"[26] Apparently, surgery was not possible, and in January 1879, in an eight-page letter from London, Nightingale wrote, "Poor Mrs. Broomhead: how patient she is: it is quite beautiful. I should like to have seen her. As she wished to see me: but I scarcely can wish her to live another year. Please tell her I always remember: & continue your kind care."[27] Five years later, Nightingale wrote, "It is astonishing how Mrs. Broomhead lives."[28]

Dunn died in 1892 at the age of fifty-six, and Nightingale engaged Dr. George Godfrey MacDonald to look after the villagers. She wrote to her nephew Shore at Lea Hurst, briefly describing the villagers and asking him to find out if they liked Dr. MacDonald. She even wanted the opinion of Sister Hannah Allen, whom she described as "insane" and as believing that the whole village wanted to poison her. She asked Shore to "Pray give her £1—Please ask her how she likes Dr. MacDonald, who attends her for me—to little purpose, I fear."[29] Nightingale continued working with the folk at Lea Hurst and, with the passing of years, many of them died. Poor Hannah Allen died in 1896.[30]

Nursing Family

Nursing ill family members was much more intimate than caring for the villagers. Nightingale's correspondence shows the extent to which she nursed her mother and her sister Parthenope. What is surprising, given her busy schedule, is the way she also took responsibility for the health of her brother-in-law Sir Harry Verney, his children by his deceased wife, their children, and Sir Harry's employees. Beginning in the 1870s, as her mother Fanny's eyesight and mental capacity began failing, Nightingale spent much time with her at Embley and organized her care. In 1872, during July, August, and September, she slept in the music room next to her mother's room so she would be there if her mother needed her. This also allowed her to watch closely the care given by Webb, the caretaker employed by the family, whom Nightingale did not trust.[31] Even though Webb did most of the physical care, Nightingale was also involved, including giving her mother the "po" (bedpan).[32] Nightingale drew up a list headed, "Measures essential *for my Mother's care*," which told family members when to see her mother and how to question Webb to make sure that the care was adequate.[33]

Nightingale's relationship with her mother deepened during the course of her mother's illness. They had wonderful conversations which Nightingale observed only arose "when she is lying quite quietly in bed . . . *never* when she is walking about. . . . Then her mind seems utterly to fail her. The most painful confusion of mind arises in which she often makes the most painful mistakes & remarks."[34]

In January 1880, Nightingale's mother took a turn for the worse. Nightingale described for Parthenope her mother's incessant cough and the inability "to get up the expectoration."[35] In a note a week later, she described "sad restlessness & dryness of mouth."[36] A few days later, on February 2, 1880, Fanny died.

Obviously, other family members besides Nightingale were involved in the mother's care. Nightingale corresponded with both Parthenope and Sir Harry about Fanny's condition and about decisions to be made about caregivers. But, as the unmarried daughter, much of the responsibility and the actual staying with her mother fell to Florence. Florence accepted the responsibility as a daughter but carried out the task with her skills as a nurse. In this instance, she both gave hands-on care and supervised the overall care. The family relied on Florence as both a daughter and a nurse. Her mother's death ended, for Nightingale, ten years of care on many levels—actual physical care, observation and planning of care, supervision of care, and consultation with family members and physicians. She had put her work in London on hold when required. For example, in December 1872, she wrote, "I left the most harassing & pressing business unfinished in London in order to come down here again."[37] Now, with both her parents gone, she was free to concentrate again on her own projects.

Within two years, however, she was involved in the same kind of care for her sister Parthenope, who had a severe arthritic condition. The correspondence about Parthenope was with Sir Harry and Margaret Verney, Sir Harry's daughter-in-law. In 1882, there was still confusion about Parthenope's diagnosis. Nightingale wrote to Sir Harry in November, "she has had 10 Doctors in little more than 5 months! Nothing could be worse hardly for her – I will gladly see Dr. Ogle or Dr. Acland if you like if a time can be found when I *can* see him, & give him a fee. He will certainly tell me the truth"[38] [original emphasis]. A month later she wrote, "I have had the Night Nurse's written report, & have had Julie [presumably a Claydon employee] for an hour. And I have written the enclosed to Dr. Ogle to be sent by you, please. If you wish Parthe to see Sir W. Gull again, please add a note to this to Dr. Ogle. I cannot say that Parthe seems better. *Unless you have heard from Dr. Acland* I propose to write *him* an account of her state" (original emphasis).[39] Although Nightingale seemed to be taking a lot of responsibility for Parthenope on herself, she clearly did nothing without consulting Sir Harry, who seems to have accepted Nightingale's help. By mid-December, Margaret Verney had come to look after Parthenope.

Nightingale still, however, directed Parthenope's care on a day-to-day basis. Nightingale informed Dr. Ogle that Margaret would henceforth "take charge of the carrying out of his orders."[40] Margaret sent records to Nightingale of Parthenope's sleep and intake of food and drink. Nightingale returned the records with further advice: the quantities eaten should be recorded, the brandy should be added to the record, Parthenope should be readied for sleep by 10 P.M., and then "nothing to be done in her room after night-*pill* at 10" (original emphasis).[41]

Late in January 1883, Nightingale wrote Margaret that Dr. Acland had visited her in London, as she thought to discuss Parthenope's condition. He said that Parthenope was improving, that "the effusion in the knee was disappearing – but that there was a 'thickening,' not implicating the joint which was troublesome to her. . . . everything would depend on 'nutrition'. . . . [and] he very much wished that she would take enemas – they were so much better for her than medicine."[42] Apparently, however, the real reason Acland had visited Nightingale was to discuss Sir Harry's physical condition. Sir Harry was in his eighties and Parthenope in her sixties. Acland had noticed "a great alteration in Sir Harry in the last 3 months . . . [changing from] a hale active old man [to] a very feeble old man." Acland believed Sir Harry to be in a vulnerable state where "a very slight illness, would carry him off." Nightingale wrote out this information for Margaret, who could then pass it on to her husband, Captain Edmund Verney, and to his brother Fred, as she saw fit. They also, obviously, saw Nightingale as the authority on her family's health. Correspondence about Sir Harry's and Parthenope's health continued until their deaths. Parthenope died in 1890 and Sir Harry in 1894.

Nightingale also nursed Sir Harry's grandchildren. One incident, in the spring of 1889, concerns the children of Sir Harry's youngest son Fred and his wife Maude. Gwendolyn, age five, and Ralph, seven, visited Claydon without their mother. Their father is not mentioned, but a Miss Shalders, referred to in the correspondence, was probably their nanny. While at Claydon, the children developed measles, Ralph first and then Gwendolyn. Ralph seems to have recovered without incident. Nightingale wrote daily reports of Gwendolyn's temperature, pulse, and cough to Maude. On June 16, temperature was 102.4, pulse 130, and cough "kept quiet by poultices." On June 17, "cough much better—(It was not a whoop but only the cough of measles)." By June 18, temperature was 98.8, pulse 86, rash fading, and cough much better. Nightingale seems to have enjoyed this little stint nursing the children. She wrote, "oh how sorry I am to leave them – God bless them."[43]

In 1890, Gwendolyn, now nine, and her seven-year-old sister Kathleen developed enlarged tonsils. Fred and Maude must have taken the children to several doctors and then become confused by their differing opinions. They then consulted Nightingale, who contacted Dr. George Ord, one of the doctors who had examined the children.[44] In all, four doctors were consulted, and Nightingale drew up a chart with four columns to aid in decision making. The first column listed the names of the doctors, the next column their findings regarding tonsils and "adenoidal vegetations," then the name of the surgeon they would recommend, and finally a column recommending for or against surgery for tonsils only or for tonsils and adenoids.[45] Nightingale had never heard about adenoidal vegetations before, and so she consulted further about that. After many letters and telegrams back and forth, the children had both tonsils and adenoids removed on November 12. The next day, after hearing of the success of the operations, Nightingale wrote, "I am singing a Te Deum in my heart as loud as I can."[46] Still later in the month, in a letter to Fred marked "PRIVATE," Nightingale wrote, "Accept my share of the expense of successfully cutting the two dear throats" (original emphasis).[47]

Although the incident of the tonsillectomies involved many letters, there was other correspondence with both Fred and Maude about projects and family matters not related to health. Nightingale had a similar relationship with Edmund and Margaret Verney and their children. When it came to health, "Aunt Florence" represented the nineteenth-century equivalent of the Web. She knew whom to consult in each case, and she eagerly accepted new knowledge and explored further.

Nursing Neighbors

In 1887, a Claydon employee, Mrs. Robertson, saw Dr. Philip Benson, the local physician, about pain in her groin. Nightingale wrote to Benson asking him to tell her, "as to an old Nurse, what exactly is the matter."[48] She heard from Benson, and there followed a series of letters between Parthenope and Nightingale arranging for Mrs. Robertson to go to London and be fitted for a truss. Nightingale described several doctors for Robertson to choose from and offered to pay the doctor's fee rather than have Mrs. Robertson attend the outpatient clinic at St. Thomas's Hospital. She arranged doctor's appointments in relation to train times and arranged Mrs. Robertson's stay in London, including taking her meals at Nightingale's home. Nightingale seemed knowledgeable about trusses, and that it took "two or three times of fitting . . . or it only ends in the Patient being miserable & having to *come up to London again*" (original emphasis).[49]

Wherever she was, Nightingale's ears and eyes were alert to physical conditions. On one occasion at Claydon House, she heard one of the maids, Emily

Baker, "breathing hard like a steam engine" as she lit the fire in the dressing room. Nightingale arranged for Baker to see Dr. Benson, who prescribed Squire's Preparation and rest. Nightingale arranged for a follow-up visit so he could check the effectiveness of the Squire's Preparation. She asked Benson "to speak to her about the 'rest'" since Baker was planning to work at her mother's lodging house. She also asked, "do you think she *laces* too tightly?" (original emphasis). Nightingale rarely saw this maid but heard her lighting the fire. She arranged a doctor's appointment and a follow-up for him to evaluate the effectiveness of his treatment. In the meantime, she discovered the maid's plans to move to her mother's lodging house. Nightingale had assessed the maid's condition, gathered further data, and arranged for consultation and treatment. She also needed to know the results of the treatment and in her letter to Benson wrote, "Perhaps you would be kind enough to write me a note afterwards."[50] Nursing employees was not something that Nightingale dabbled in. She carried the process to completion.

Just as Nightingale worked with Dr. Dunn at Lea Hurst, so she worked with Dr. Benson at Claydon. There must have been an underlying agreement with Sir Harry about nursing his employees. In any case, Nightingale herself paid Dr. Benson.[51] In December 1888, Nightingale sent a progress report to Benson on Elizabeth Hubbard, a young Lea Hurst under-housemaid whom Nightingale brought to Claydon. Hubbard had two problems, one related to her monthly period and the other an enlarged goiter. For menstruation, she was given iron and ergot of rye. Nightingale reported that Hubbard's monthly period came on, and that the iron had not made her bowels "costive." She only took "opening medicine" (laxative) once. Nightingale reported that the girl "looks more lively and the goiter has sensibly diminished and is a great deal softer and less stiff."[52] A year later, Nightingale reported to Benson again. Elizabeth Hubbard's goiter had been measured every fortnight and remained "exactly the same."[53]

Nightingale juggled many projects at once. She was corresponding with Dunn about the villagers and employees at Lea Hurst and with Benson and other doctors about the Claydon employees, and she was also writing to Sir Harry, to the Duke of Devonshire through Sir Harry, to Georgina Hurt, and to Bonham Carter about the Buxton Hospital.

Nursing in Hospitals

In 1878, Nightingale became aware that the nursing care of bedridden patients in the Devonshire Hospital at Buxton was "abominable." This was of particular concern to her because it was here that Dr. Dunn admitted the villagers and cottagers for whom she and Dunn were caring. It seemed useless to send these patients to a hospital that worsened their conditions. She was, after all, paying "10/a week" for each of her patients admitted to Buxton Hospital[54] and had a right to know that they were receiving good care. She solicited reports about the care given there to her patients and discovered, for example, that there was no night nurse and that severely rheumatic patients were left all night without being moved or given bedpans. The patients were discouraged from waking the nurse for care at night and were, in fact, "in bodily fear of the management."[55] There was neglect in feeding patients and in protecting them from cold drafts. Some of Nightingale's information came from Mrs. Limb, widow of the local stonemason. Nightingale paid for her admission to Buxton Hospital for severe rheumatism. Mrs. Limb was put in a ward with five other helpless patients who were left all night without care. One woman was left all night on the commode, unable to get into bed. Mrs. Limb finally had a friend bring her home.[56] Nightingale felt so responsible for what had happened to Mrs. Limb that she spent £60 a year providing medical and nursing care and assistive appliances for her. Mrs. Limb died with the greatest suffering at younger than fifty years of age. Nightingale later believed she should have prosecuted the hospital. These findings about Buxton Hospital, not surprisingly, set Nightingale's reform instinct into high gear. She nursed the villagers by correspondence; she also worked at reforming the nursing they received at Buxton Hospital at a distance.

Buxton Hospital was the nearest hospital to the villages of Lea and Holloway. This whole area, on the edge of the beautiful Peaks District, contains many hot springs. Buxton became a spa area before the hospital was built. In 1779, the Buxton Bath Charity was formed, and in the mid-1850s, charity patients were accommodated in private lodgings not always convenient to the baths. In the early 1860s, through the auspices of the Sixth Duke of Devonshire, a charity hospital was established, with surgical and accident wards added later. Subsequent dukes continued their interest in the hospital and served on the hospital board.[57]

Nightingale began her attempts at reform in a low-key way, what she described as working "with quietness and caution."[58] Looking back later, she believed her early attempts at reforming Buxton Hospital had failed because she had been "over prudent, owing to the fear of injuring the Patients who were there."[59] On November 3, 1878, she asked Dr. Dunn to help her find someone to discreetly look into the situation, and on November 4, she asked Sir Harry Verney to find a lady to make an enquiry.[60] Miss Georgina Hurt, who was or became a friend of Parthenope, took on the job and provided Nightingale with "fresh & fresh abominations," including the fact that some of the ladies approached for the enquiry knew the conditions were bad and had done nothing to change them.[61] On January 2, 1879, Nightingale reported to Dr. Dunn, "I have set on foot an enquiry into that abominable place. The Master & Mistress are leaving (drunk)."[62] She described the master and mistress (i.e., steward and matron) as coming from a workhouse milieu and running Buxton Hospital as though it were a workhouse, with any patient care being given by other patients. Because the patients with severe rheumatism were in a room by themselves, there were no convalescent patients to help them.

The dismissal of the matron and steward was just a beginning and did nothing to provide care to bedridden patients at night. Nightingale decided to enlist a more powerful ally, the Duke of Devonshire. She appealed to the duke through Sir Harry, a Member of Parliament and a member of the Nightingale Fund, which operated Nightingale's School of Nursing at St. Thomas' Hospital.[63] There followed a flurry of letters among these three participants in a round-robin fashion: Nightingale writing to Sir Harry, Sir Harry writing to the duke and enclosing the Nightingale letters, the duke writing to Sir Harry, and Sir Harry writing to Nightingale and enclosing the duke's letters. Some of Nightingale's letters were marked "private and confidential," and she specified which could be forwarded to the duke. Sir Harry met with Nightingale, and finally even the duke visited Nightingale when he was in London.

In the beginning, Nightingale had qualms about the ability of the duke to carry out the enquiry. She wrote to Sir Harry, "I am such an old 'hand' & know what blunders may be made by the best intentions not practically acquainted with Hospital Nursing."[64] She worried that he was not a "practical man"[65] and in fact that he was "a little unreasonable."[66] After she met the duke, however, she reported, "the D. of D. very satisfactory: sure he means to do his best: very shy: quite affectionate, particularly when speaking of Sir Harry: very straight to the point." She concluded, nonetheless, "I'm not sure Buxton Hospital won't be too many for him."[67] Part of Nightingale's concern was that she wanted the duke to appear to be acting on his own, without using her name.[68] Nightingale had good reason to request anonymity because she knew that her name would cause a stir, a stir that she described in 1856 as "the buz fuz which is about my name."[69] She recognized that if her name were used, "the Hospital books will be examined: & the names of Patients whom I have had there will be ascertained. It will then become a question of proving or disproving the statement of this or that Patient – which, I submit, is just the thing to be avoided, if you wish to arrive at the truth."[70] She was concerned about the repercussions on Dr. Dunn who needed to make a living, and she also surmised that using her name would actually hinder the duke's inquiry. She believed that the duke himself making inquiries would strengthen the case.

Nightingale wanted the total nursing to be examined, not particular complaints. To this end, she supplied Sir Harry with a questionnaire for the duke to use in his inquiry. This included questions about the number of nurses, their training, their duties to the patients, their supervision, and their pay; about the matron, her training, and her duties; about the hospital and the number and types of wards.[71] In seeking this kind of information, the duke would be acting appropriately for his position as patron of the hospital and would not be reporting and investigating specific complaints.

At some point in April 1879, however, the managers at Buxton Hospital must have become aware that it was under scrutiny. In a clever move, Joseph Taylor, secretary of Buxton Hospital, applied to Mrs. Wardroper, the matron at St. Thomas' Hospital, for nursing staff. This would circumvent the whole enquiry. Nightingale bewailed it as a "movement to turn our flank."[72] This occasioned another great flurry of letters and brought Henry Bonham Carter into the situation. Bonham Carter was Nightingale's cousin and secretary of the Nightingale Fund and would be involved if trained nurses were sent from St. Thomas's. Nightingale proclaimed Taylor "quite a common sort of man," and "an ordinary, vulgar, uneducated clerk."[73] She pointed out to Bonham Carter the ignorance Taylor had shown about his own hospital.

This was the quandary: if the Nightingale School of Nursing at St. Thomas's Hospital immediately sent a head nurse with four other nurses as requested, Nightingale would have to stop the enquiry *and* these new nurses would have to work within the awful situation at Buxton. If, however, they refused to send nurses, Buxton Hospital would hire untrained nurses and perpetuate the poor nursing. After consulting with Sir Harry and Georgina Hurt, Nightingale suggested to Bonham Carter that "he should not say anything *at all like declining*, but merely write *a vague reply, putting it off*" (emphasis original).[74] This would allow them the possibility of taking over the nursing at Buxton Hospital after the inquiry was completed, the prospect of which Nightingale said, "warms my heart." Of course, because this was a private inquiry and Nightingale was not to be seen as involved, Mrs. Wardroper could not be given this inside information. On May 10, 1879, Nightingale informed Sir Harry that the Buxton Hospital had also applied for a head nurse to the Devonshire Square Nursing Sisters, "who are nothing but untrained private Nurses." Nightingale was afraid that Buxton would hire untrained nurses and then tell the Duke of Devonshire "that everything was put right."[75]

But where was the Duke of Devonshire in all this, and should he be told what was happening? Nightingale consulted with both Miss Georgina Hurt and Sir Harry, who both strongly advised against informing the duke. Nightingale believed the move by Buxton Hospital was the result of something the duke had done, and that "it would be a pity to traverse him."[76] At the same time, she was uneasy about not informing him.

The inquiry instigated by Nightingale seems to have discovered some surprises. In a letter to Dr. Dunn later in the 1880s, Nightingale recounted an incident uncovered during the inquiry at Buxton Hospital. Apparently, at some point before the inquiry, Nightingale had paid for hospital admission for Charles Walters and was later informed that he had been discharged with his condition unchanged. Actually, Walters was dying and, in fact, died. As Nightingale noted, it was by "the merest accident" that the person who paid the patient's hospital costs was also the "one who instituted an enquiry."[77] She wondered how often deaths went unreported. Nightingale also blamed the nursing at Buxton for the death of widow Limb, who never recovered from her stay at the hospital. Nightingale wrote, "I have her quite on my conscience . . . I am afraid it is that abominable no-nursing at Buxton which has made her worse."

Here are some of the findings of the inquiry.[78] There was a lady housekeeper and a head nurse, "separate authorities, without any concurrence or system." Nightingale described the circuitous history that brought this about as "strange & sad." A Miss Smith elected as Lady Superintendent of Nurses was "blamed for 'creating an animus' against a drunken Master & Matron," who were then dismissed. Miss Smith was then "denounced as having been accessory to the dismissal of those two deserving Officers, the drinking Master & Matron." To replace the master and matron, a lady housekeeper, Mrs. Russell, was hired but given no description of her duties or authority. Consequently, there was trouble between the housekeeper and the lady superintendent. Then the lady superintendent was dismissed for "impropriety, if not immorality, with the '***House Surgeon***,' . . . contrary to all instructions." Nightingale commented wryly, "*When is it **according** to instructions*" (emphasis original).[79] It would seem that a head nurse was hired to replace the improper lady superintendent. And, no, the house surgeon was not dismissed for this; the hospital simply "feared" that they might have to get rid of him.

Through the inquiry, Nightingale also learned that there were four untrained nurses with twenty-six patients to each nurse. Later she reported that "the 'full staff' consists, it is said, of 'Head Nurse' (trained), 2 *trained* Nurses (not trained)? 1 to the Male, 1 to the Female side, & 4 Probationers *to 158 beds!!*" (emphasis original). Nightingale concluded that there was no authority over anyone. She believed what was needed was "one *female* head" to be in charge of "all the *Nursing & domestic* arrangements." This person was "to see that the Nurses *Strictly carry out the orders of the Medical Staff*: without this there can be no Nursing." Nightingale continued conferring with Bonham Carter and the Duke (emphasis original).[80]

On May 20, 1879, Nightingale asked Bonham Carter for his recommendations for Buxton Hospital, which she would send on to the Duke of Devonshire.

The duke had been involved in investigating problems at the hospital; now he could concern himself with correcting those problems. The duke had asked for "a short paper,' saying '*what we recommend for the future rather than finding fault with the past.*'" The duke had arranged to visit Nightingale, and he wanted this information before he came. He also explained to Nightingale that, although there were problems at the hospital, it "does much good." He had also wisely stated that "*we can work only with the material we have: the people*" (emphasis original). Nightingale planned that she and the duke would then "talk it out."[81] Bonham Carter replied that there had been insufficient communication for making specific recommendations and they should wait to appoint a properly qualified matron.[82]

Some improvements were made, possibly by actions of the Duke of Devonshire. On November 8, 1879, Nightingale thanked Dr. Dunn for his work in improving the care at Buxton Hospital. She stated, "I conclude that you are satisfied that the Nursing for *helpless* Patients is now what it ought to be. For, if you remember, persons who were able to shift for themselves were very well satisfied with their treatment, even while the bed-ridden ones were suffering the abominations we know of. And the person who gives his name to the Hospital [the Duke of Devonshire] told me distinctly this when I appealed to him in London" (emphasis original).[83] On January 10, 1880, she again recorded her joy that the nursing had improved and asked about the new matron.

In December 1881, however, Nightingale was still soliciting information to evaluate the results of the inquiry. It seems that Georgina Hurt was staying with Parthenope. Nightingale wrote to Parthenope describing poor widow Limb's experience and requesting that Hurt write to tell her "what she considers the present state of the Nursing, the Matronship & management" of Buxton Hospital.[84]

Nightingale's work to reform the nursing at Buxton Hospital is at once an example of the traditional role of a woman helping her neighbors, a wealthy middle-class woman providing for the lower classes, and, at the same time, a skilled professional using her knowledge and resources to reform a poorly functioning institution. This Buxton situation presents a microcosm through which to examine Nightingale as a woman of power and influence. Women of power disturb the peace and may not be welcomed by others in power. Nightingale obviously knew that as soon as her name was known, tension and defensiveness would result. Actually, she routinely avoided having her name used for projects.[85] Even though she was paying patient fees at the Buxton Hospital, Nightingale had no authority in that hospital. She began softly, with the purpose of collecting information. She was not a busybody meddler dashing in with complaints, even if they were legitimate complaints.

Nightingale had the big picture in mind, and she was working for reform of the nursing system. For her, there was no nursing if there was not a nursing system. She soon found that walking softly, using women without influence or authority, was limited in its effectiveness in gathering data. And, although Dr. Dunn was involved in the collaboration to improve the nursing, Nightingale was considerate in her expectations of him. She got information from him but did not press him to take any action. She was conscious that his living depended on his medical practice, and she would not jeopardize that. It was at this point that she enlisted the aid of the Duke of Devonshire. It was the influence of her name, of course, and her family connections that brought the duke on board. Reform of the nursing at Buxton Hospital was successful to a point. Although the system had not completely changed and there were still staff problems, helpless patients were being nursed both at night and during the day. This indicates that, with the dismissal of the matron and steward, the hospital was no longer functioning on a workhouse model. Nightingale's reform at Buxton Hospital was an integral part of her nursing of the villagers. She was managing their care, and that management extended to wherever they were receiving care and to whoever was giving the care.

Even the brief examples given of Nightingale's nursing care of villagers, family, and employees, selected from hundreds of letters, provide overwhelming evidence of Nightingale's ongoing nursing activity. Her skill at soliciting pertinent information about the patients and using the information to arrange appropriate care was demonstrated repeatedly. That care often included referral to a physician. However, she also, on occasion, gave hands-on physical care and always requested information about the results of the care.

One may quickly dismiss the accusation that Nightingale was impulsive and that her work with the cottagers around Lea Hurst was an "impulsive venture." Her nursing of these individuals was sustained over many years and deliberative. These letters, in addition, provide a picture of Nightingale as a warm, down-to-earth, caring person. The Buxton Hospital situation suggests that she had no interest in wielding power for her own enhancement but did so simply to further her cause in nursing.

JOYCE SCHROEDER MACQUEEN, BN, MED, MSc.
Associate Professor (Retired)
Laurentian University
5627 Clearwater Lake Road
Sudbury, ON P3G 1L9, Canada

Acknowledgments

I thank Associated Medical Services, Inc., for funding that made research for this article possible, and The Collected Works of Florence Nightingale Project for the wealth of materials made available to me.

Notes

1. F.B. Smith, *Florence Nightingale: Reputation and Power* (London: Croom Helm, 1982), 18.
2. Sue M. Goldie, ed., *Florence Nightingale: Letters from the Crimea 1854–1856* (Manchester, UK: Mandolin, 1997), 4.
3. Martha Vicinus and Bea Nergaard, eds., *Ever Yours, Florence Nightingale: Selected Letters* (London: Virago Press, 1989), 5.
4. Florence Nightingale to Reverend Mother Mary Clare Moore, March 28, 1856, Nightingale Collection, Wellcome Institute for the History of Medicine MSS 8996/37 (hereafter NC, Wellcome). The "extras" were special additions to the regular diet.
5. Florence Nightingale, *Notes on Nursing* (London: Harrison and Sons, 1859). Emphasis throughout is original unless otherwise noted.
6. Nightingale, *Notes,* 20.
7. Nightingale to Julia Ann Elizabeth Roundell, August 4, 1896, Nightingale Collection, British Library ADD MSS 45,813/219v (hereafter NC, BL).
8. Nightingale to Victoria Adelaide Mary Louise, Princess Royal and wife of Frederick III, German Emperor, Letter in pencil, circa 1872, NC, BL ADD MSS 45,750, f 48.
9. Nightingale to Louisa Mary Elizabeth, wife of Frederick William Louis, Grand Duke of Baden, draft of a letter, March 1879, NC, BL ADD MSS 45,750, f163v.
10. S. Lees, *Handbook for Hospital Sisters*, ed. Henry W. Acland (London, 1874).
11. Tom Olson and Eileen Walsh, *Handling the Sick: The Women of St. Luke's and the Nature of Nursing, 1892–1937* (Columbus: The Ohio State University Press, 2004), 94.
12. Gillian Gill, *Nightingales: The Extraordinary Upbringing and Curious Life of Miss Florence Nightingale* (New York: Ballantine, 2004), 152, 177.
13. Gill, *Nightingales,* 191, 214.
14. Barbara Montgomery Dossey, *Florence Nightingale: Mystic, Visionary, Healer* (Springhouse, PA: Springhouse, 2000), 296.
15. For information on The Collected Works of Florence Nightingale Project, see http://www.sociology.uoguelph.ca/fnightingale/
16. Gertrude Himmelfarb, *The De-Moralization of Society from Victorian Virtues to Modern Values* (New York: Knopf, 1995), 149.
17. Dossey, *Florence Nightingale,* 30.
18. Nightingale to Fred Verney, June 23, 1879, NC, BL ADD MSS 68,882, f99v. Direct quotes are given as Nightingale wrote them, including phraseology, punctuation, and spelling. Italics are used for Nightingale's underlining.

19. Nightingale to Fred Verney, November 25, 1881, Nightingale Collection, London Metropolitan Archives, Florence Nightingale Museum, f45 (hereafter NC, LMA).

20. Nightingale to Dr. C.B.N. Dunn, March 24, 1879, Nightingale Collection, Derbyshire Record Office, f37 (hereafter NC, DRO).

21. Nightingale to Dr. Dunn, October 27, 1876, NC, DRO f1.

22. Nightingale to Dr. Dunn, August 22, 1877, NC, DRO f4.

23. Nightingale to Dr. Dunn, August 23, 1877, NC, DRO f5.

24. Nightingale to Dr. Dunn, September 3, 1878, NC, DRO f21.

25. Nightingale to Dr. Dunn, September 12, 1878, NC, DRO f19.

26. Nightingale to Dr. Dunn, October 5, 1878, NC, DRO f23.

27. Nightingale to Dr. Dunn, January 21, 1879, NC, DRO f33av.

28. Nightingale to Dr. Dunn, July 22, 1884, NC, DRO f78.

29. Nightingale to Shore Smith, n.d., NC, BL ADD MSS 45,795, f144r. From notes in pencil that seem to be an enclosure for a letter to Shore Smith. The date must be after Dunn's death in 1892.

30. Nightingale to Mr. Yeomans, March 6, 1896, Royal College of Nurses FN 1/22/2.

31. Nightingale to ?, December 17, 1872, NC, Wellcome MSS 9005/170.

32. Nightingale to Parthenope Verney, March 7, 1873, NC, Wellcome MSS 9006/25.

33. Nightingale to ?, December 7, 1872, NC, Wellcome MSS 9005 letter 170.

34. Nightingale to ?, n.d., NC, Wellcome MSS 9004 letter/draft 50 marked Private.

35. Nightingale to Parthenope Verney, January 24, 1880, NC, Wellcome MSS 9008/3.

36. Nightingale to Parthenope Verney? January 30, 1880, NC, Wellcome MSS 9008/5.

37. Nightingale to ?, December 17, 1872, NC, Wellcome MSS 9005/170.

38. Nightingale to Sir Harry Verney, Novermber 6, 1882, NC, Wellcome 9009/104.

39. Nightingale to Sir Harry, December 12, 1882, NC, Wellcome 9009/127.

40. Nightingale to Dr. Ogle, December 15, 1882, NC, Wellcome 9009/133.

41. Nightingale to Margaret Verney, December 15, 1882, January 2, 1883, January 5, 1883, NC, Wellcome 9009/148, also 133, 151.

42. Nightingale to Margaret Verney, January 27, 1883, NC, Wellcome 9009/161 marked "private."

43. Nightingale to Maude Verney, June 16, 1886, June 17, 1886, June 18, 1886, NC, BL ADD, MSS 68,884, f52, f54, f56.

44. Nightingale to Fred Verney, November 9, 1890, NC, BL ADD MSS 68,886, ff143–5.

45. Nightingale to Fred Verney, November 9, 1890, NC, BL ADD MSS 68,886, f159.

46. Nightingale to Fred Verney, November 9, 1890, NC, BL ADD MSS 68,886, f171.

47. Nightingale to Fred Verney, November 9, 1890, NC, BL ADD MSS 68,886, f180.

48. Nightingale to Dr. Philip Benson, September 7, 1887, Columbia UC-180.

49. Nightingale to Parthenope Verney, September 10 & 13, 1887, NC, Wellcome MSS 9011/174, 175.

50. Nightingale to Dr. Benson, September 26, 1888, NC, Wellcome MSS 9012/55.

51. Nightingale to Dr. Benson, November 25, 1889, NC, Wellcome MSS 9012/25.

52. Nightingale to Dr. Benson, December 19, 1888, NC, Wellcome MSS 9012/68.

53. Nightingale to Dr. Benson, November 25, 1889, NC, Wellcome MSS 9012/252.

54. Nightingale to Sir Harry Verney, April 24, 1879, NC, Wellcome MSS 9007/219.

55. Nightingale to Sir Harry Verney, April 5, 1879, NC, Wellcome MSS 9007/198.

56. Nightingale to Parthenope Verney, December 14, 1881, NC, Wellcome MSS 9008/186.

57. www.derby.ac.uk/devonshire/history/Timeline.htm: The current Duke of Devonshire is working to have the hospital building (called the Devonshire Royal Hospital since 1934) and other surrounding buildings preserved as a heritage site.

58. Nightingale to Dr. C.B.N. Dunn, November 3, 1878, NC, DRO f 33bv.

59. Nightingale to Sir Harry Verney, April 5, 1879, NC, Wellcome MSS 9007/198.

60. Nightingale to Dr. Dunn, November 3, 1878, NC, DRO f 30–30v; Nightingale to Sir Harry Verney, November 4, 1878, NC, Wellcome MSS 9007/172.

61. Nightingale to ?, April 24, 1879, 6 A.M., NC, BL ADD MSS 47,720, F 8.

62. Nightingale to Dr. Dunn, January 2, 1879, NC, DRO f 32a.

63. Nightingale to Sir Harry Verney, April 5, 1879, NC, Wellcome MSS 9007/198.

64. Nightingale to Sir Harry Verney, April 12, 1879, NC, DRO f 36av.

65. Nightingale to Sir Harry Verney, April 18, 1879, NC, Wellcome MSS 9007/216.

66. Nightingale to Sir Harry Verney, May 21, 1879, NC, Wellcome MSS 9007/236.

67. Nightingale to Sir Harry Verney, May 27, 1879, NC, Wellcome MSS 9007/237.

68. Nightingale to Sir Harry Verney, April 12,1879, NC, DRO f 36a.

69. Nightingale to ?, n.d., but probably August 1856, NC, BL ADD MSS 45,796, f 71.

70. Nightingale to Sir Harry Verney, April 18, 1879, NC, Wellcome MSS 9007/214.

71. Nightingale to Sir Harry Verney, April 5, 1879, NC, Wellcome MSS 9007/198.

72. Nightingale to Sir Harry Verney, April 24, 1879, NC, Wellcome MSS 9007/219.

73. Nightingale to Henry Bonham Carter, April 28, 1879, NC, BL ADD MSS 47,720, f 14; Nightingale to ?, April 24, 1879, 6 A.M., NC, BL ADD MSS 47,720, F 8.

74. Nightingale to Henry Bonham Carter, April 28, 1879, NC, BL ADD MSS 47,720, f 15.

75. Nightingale to Sir Harry Verney, May 10, 1879, NC, Wellcome MSS 9007/229.

76. Nightingale to Henry Bonham Carter, April 28, 1879, NC, BL ADD MSS 47,720, ff 14–15.

77. Nightingale to probably Dr. Dunn, likely 1885, NC, BL ADD MSS RP 2055, jumbled pages, follows report of Gordon's death at Khartoum.

78. Nightingale to ?, pencil draft, May 14, 1879, NC, BL ADD MSS 47,720, ff 25–31.

79. Nightingale to ?, pencil draft, May 14, 1879, BL MSS ADD 47,720, f28. Use of both italics and bold signifies double underlining in the original.

80. Nightingale to ?, pencil draft, May 14, 1879, NC, BL ADD MSS 47,720, ff 25–31.

81. Nightingale to probably Henry Bonham Carter, initialed draft, May 20, 1879, NC, BL ADD MSS 47,720, f 32.

82. Henry Bonham Carter to Nightingale, May 20, 1879, NC, BL ADD MSS 47,720, f 33.

83. Nightingale to Dr. Dunn, November 8, 1879, NC, DRO f 50.

84. Nightingale to Parthenope Verney, December 14, 1881, NC Wellcome MSS 9008/186.

85. Nightingale, *The Collected Works of Florence Nightingale,* ed. Lynn McDonald, vol. 1, *Florence Nightingale: An Introduction to Life and Family* (Waterloo, Ontario, Canada: Wilfrid Laurier University Press, 2001), 42.

The Nursing Radicalism of the Honourable Albinia Brodrick, 1861–1955

ANN WICKHAM
Dublin City University

The Honourable Albinia Brodrick was born into the English aristocracy in 1861 but died a pauper in Ireland in 1955. During her lifetime, she moved from England to Ireland, changed her name from Albinia Brodrick to Gobnait Ni Bhruadair, and embraced Irish nationalist ideals that were in total opposition to the unionist political beliefs of her family. Throughout all these changes, this article argues, her life, work, and ideals were shaped by her embrace of the profession of nursing and her commitment to the rights of nurses. Her dedication and energy helped shape nursing politics in Ireland in the early twentieth century.

Brodrick was born on December 17, 1861, in Middlesex, England, to William Brodrick, Viscount Middleton, and his wife Augusta. She had the usual upbringing and activities of an aristocratic Protestant daughter, including attending concerts and balls at Buckingham Palace.[1] She became familiar with politics as she accompanied her father on his visits to the House of Lords. She also accompanied him on visits to the family estates in County Cork, Ireland.[2] However, there was always more to Brodrick than the ritualistic rounds of the upper classes. At the end of her twenties, she was known to be writing articles on political and scientific issues for English journals and possibly lived in Oxford as hostess for her uncle, George C. Brodrick, Warden (1831–1903) of Merton College.[3] Yet, these activities were obviously not enough for her. By 1904, she had become a nurse.

Her introduction to nursing was not easy. She trained as a certificated nurse at the District Infirmary in Ashton-under-Lyne, and in later life, she was to refer to the hardships she experienced in her role as a nursing superintendent in a workhouse.[4] By 1909, she was able to declare that she was "a trained nurse; I have the certificate of a trained midwife; I have the certificate of a health visitor, and I have two certificates to qualify me as a sanitary inspector."[5]

Nursing History Review 15 (2007): 51–64. A publication of the American Association for the History of Nursing. Copyright © 2007 Springer Publishing Company.

Brodrick and Ireland

In 1904, at the age of forty-two, Brodrick moved to Ireland but not to the estates of her family. She not only did her midwifery training in Dublin in 1905 but also spent some time in Kerry learning Irish. In 1908, she purchased land at West Cove near Caherdaniel in Kerry in the west of Ireland. The poverty of the land can be gauged by the fact that it was in one of the areas covered by the Congested Districts Board, an institution established by the British government to attempt to promote development in areas that were overpopulated or "congested" and where the population was regarded as permanently close to starving.[6] This was to be her home for the rest of her life, although the next twenty years saw her traveling continually between England and Ireland.

Appalled by the poverty she saw, and in particular by the health problems of the population, Brodrick set about building a hospital using her own money. She wrote to readers of the *British Journal of Nursing* on the evolution of her ideas and of her desire in middle age to build "A Hospital for Kerry, for one corner of Kerry, because of the children haunted by tuberculosis, the women tortured in childbirth, the men struck low before their time." She had received little encouragement for this idea when she sought advice on her scheme and she castigated those who derided her plans, asking, "Did *you* ever need to be driven eighteen miles with a fractured thigh? Has *your* wife bled to death in childbirth for want of help? Is it *your* child that goes lame for life for want of treatment?"[7]

Brodrick called her scheme Ballincoona, the House of Help, and from the start it was no modest undertaking. Four acres were reclaimed from bog, 5,000 trees were planted, a road was laid, and a twenty-foot well was dug. A shelter, a storehouse, a workshop, a fowl house, a piggery, and a cattle house were all completed and the foundations for the hospital laid in the first year, all for an expenditure of £2,620. In this initiative, she did not break with her upper-class background but rather used her background to support her schemes. She especially used her social contacts to raise financial support for her interests and commitments, "explaining, upbraiding, cajoling, pleading, warning, exhorting."[8] Alongside the hospital, she set up a Co-operative Shop and a Cooperative Agricultural Society whose members would work together and reap the profits of their labors rather than see them going to an owner. She hoped that such developments would help stop emigration and assist the local population.[9]

This scheme, with its grand beginnings, was to be a central concern in Brodrick's life, but the extensive nature of her ambitions was to cause her enormous difficulties. By September 1911, the walls of the hospital were up, the majority of the windows glazed, and the slating of the roof three-fourths finished, but she was already anticipating that her plans could be brought to a standstill through lack of funds.[10] Her income was not sufficient to support her dream. The cooperative was not a drain and did in fact increase in business. But, despite disposing of her investments, selling her furniture, undertaking paid literary work, giving lectures, and writing begging letters to members of the aristocracy, she still faced the problem of money for the hospital. By 1912, she had exhausted her own finances. She had built the hospital but was unable to finish and open it. "I have done my utmost, living the simplest of simple lives in my tiny farm cottage upon about 5s a week. I have sold my beautiful old furniture, my china, knick knacks and jewellery, but still we cannot get sufficient money and I am obliged to beg ... the lack of money fetters us continually".[11]

She visited the United States in the autumn of that year, seeking money to continue her work, especially from Irish Americans and fellow nurses, including Lavinia Dock.[12] In the summer of 1913, enough funds having been gathered, work started again at Ballincoona. The cooperative was proceeding well and had an annual income of more than £3,000. Masons and carpenters were at work, and the hospital was finally ready for operation in time to be offered to the British government for the wounded of World War I, the whole scheme having cost more than £11,000.[13] Her offer was accepted "if and when required." However, she was notified by the British War Office in 1915 that it would not be needed,[14] and the hospital appears to have never become operational despite its imposing size. This want of progress can only be put down to the change in political beliefs Brodrick embraced at the age of fifty-four, following the 1916 rebellion in Dublin.

The Easter Rising of 1916 was an abortive attempt by some Irish nationalists to use violence to free Ireland from the system of rule by a Parliament in London. The Rising, mainly in Dublin, was quickly suppressed and was not regarded as having a lot of support among the general populace. However, this situation changed when on the orders of the British Cabinet fifteen of the leaders of the rising were quickly executed, one of the most notorious deaths being that of trade unionist James Connolly, who was shot tied to a chair because he was injured and unable to stand. The executions are regarded as marking a change in Irish opinion, a swing in favor of what had previously been a small nationalist party, Sinn Féin (Ourselves Alone).

Sinn Féin developed into a republican party committed to achieving self-rule for Ireland and the establishment of an Irish Republic. The party won most of the Irish seats in the British parliamentary election of 1918, but the winners, rather than taking their seats in London, established their own Irish parliament, Dail Eireann. In January 1919, they proclaimed an Irish Republic.

A bitter Anglo-Irish war followed, culminating in the partition of Ireland and the creation of an Irish Free State (within the British Empire and not a

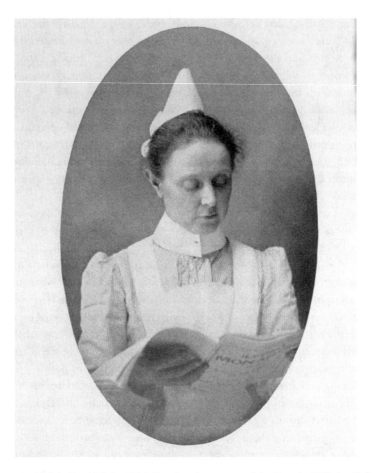

Figure 1. Albinia Brodrick in 1904. Reprinted courtesy of the Board of Trinity College Dublin.

Republic) through a treaty in December 1921. This treaty split Irish nationalists, and politics in Ireland became focused around pro- and anti-treaty positions from then on. A Civil War broke out, and some who had fought on the same side in the War for Independence now found themselves on opposing sides. The guerrilla campaign was particularly bitter in County Kerry, where Brodrick lived. There were atrocities on both sides, and many of those supporting the anti-treaty position were imprisoned. The Civil War ended in 1923, with the continued existence of a twenty-six-county Irish Free State.

Brodrick was deeply affected by these developments. She became an Irish nationalist and a member of Sinn Féin. She expressed virulently anti-British sentiments, and her republican anti-treaty politics were to shape her commitments for the rest of her life.

Brodrick and Nursing

While building Ballincoona hospital, setting up and managing the cooperative, and continually seeking funds for it, Brodrick had at the same time become active in nursing politics in both England and Ireland. Her activities took two major forms: an active role in the struggle for training and state registration for nurses and a public raising of the issues related to venereal disease. In both activities, she had an eminent profile. It was not uncommon in this period for women of rank, social class, and education who became certificated nurses to find themselves rapidly advanced to high-ranking posts and regarded as nursing leaders. Brodrick's commitment to Kerry meant that she did not take up a hospital position, but she did become a prominent writer and speaker on nursing issues.

In 1907, Brodrick joined the Society for the State Registration of Trained Nurses.[15] The need for regulation of the nursing profession was a concern of many nursing leaders in Britain and Ireland. They looked for a way to define and identify those who were fit to practice as "nurses." Referring back to the Parliamentary Act of 1858, which had established statutory registration of medical practitioners in Britain, they sought similar registration for nursing, with the title "nurse" used only by certificated nurses from identified training schools duly registered as such. In doing this, they were seeking to have members of the embryonic profession recognized as distinct from those who used the title "nurse" but were untrained, badly trained, or regarded as at a level of domestic servants.

There was to be a long struggle to achieve the goal of state registration. One of the major figures in the fight was Ethel Bedford Fenwick, founder of the British Nurses' Association and the Matrons' Council of Great Britain and Ireland and first president of the International Council of Nurses. At the end of the nineteenth century, there had already been divisions between those who supported a nonstatutory voluntary register and the faction, led by Bedford Fenwick, who sought a statutory register. Throughout the period up until 1919, when the issue was finally resolved, there were continual activities around the question of registration and bitter fights between supporters and opponents. A House of Commons Select Committee was established to consider the registration of nurses, and its 1904 report set out a persuasive case for registration.

But the government took no action, and a number of private member bills in Parliament in the following years were also unsuccessful.

In joining the Society for State Registration, Brodrick was committing herself to the fight for examination, certification, and statutory registration of nurses. By 1908, she was a delegate from that society to the National Council of Nurses.[16] As a member of the council, she became Chief Steward for the International Council of Nurses Congress to be held in 1909. She and Dock proposed and had adopted plans for a session at the congress on "Morality in Relation to Health," which Bedford Fenwick intimated would be "the most important Session of the whole Congress."[17]

Brodrick's role at the conference, particularly her support for state registration, was so outstanding that it was referred to for years to come.[18] As a member of the aristocracy, she was far from overawed by attacks on the nursing profession, particularly by the Honorable Sydney Holland, later Viscount Knutsford, an outspoken opponent of state registration for nurses.[19] She publicly cast doubt on the general accuracy of his opinions before attacking his stance on registration.[20]

Brodrick's paper on venereal disease, "Morality in Relation to Public Health," also made a major impact. She was greeted with a storm of applause at this, the first occasion when a public appeal was made for instruction on the dangers of venereal disease. A later commentator was to say, "It required courage to broach the subject of venereal diseases in those days, for the taboo of silence was almost complete, and although nurses came in contact in hospital wards with these diseases in their infectious stages they received no instructions as to protecting themselves from infection. Miss Brodrick broke down the silence."[21]

Brodrick noted the "scant instruction" given to most nurses on venereal diseases. She called for more knowledge so nurses could protect themselves in the course of their work, as well as protect and educate others. She was particularly concerned with what she saw as the innocent, the wives and children of infected men who themselves were then infected. Although Brodrick recognized that many "good and self denying women" were already attempting to deal with prostitution and its association with venereal diseases, she felt that these women, too, in many cases had little knowledge of sexually transmitted diseases.[22]

The call for knowledge enunciated by Brodrick was based on a belief that attempts to prevent venereal disease by regulation had failed.[23] In this, she was voicing for the first time in a public nursing arena the concerns and calls for reform that were beginning to be made elsewhere. Little wonder, then, that when the National Council formed a committee on the issue, at the urging of Dock and the International Council of Nurses, Brodrick was elected chairman. She continued lecturing and publishing throughout the year on both venereal disease and the need for state registration of trained nurses. By the end of the year, the strain of dealing with issues at Ballincoona led her to resign her post as chair of the committee, but she continued writing and publishing articles on the same themes.[24]

Active as she was with both her own concerns in Kerry and her active defense of the need for training and registration, Brodrick also joined in developments in Ireland. She joined the Irish Nurses Association, established in 1904, which supported the movement for state registration. In June 1913, the association organized the first annual nursing conference and exhibition in Dublin for the National Council of Trained Nurses of Great Britain and Ireland. As one of the vice presidents of the conference, Brodrick had a high profile and again took a leading action when she raised the issue of venereal disease with her paper "Black Plague, or Venereal Disease."[25] In addition, Brodrick pursued her arguments for the need for training and registration in an Irish context. She took up her pen against the United Irishwomen, a women's group concerned with the health of the rural poor, when she thought they were going to introduce an untrained nurse into a rural area.[26] She argued that untrained nurses "were cheating the poor, and blocking legislation for better workers," and called again for training and registration.[27]

Brodrick's concern and activities in relation to the need for training and registration intensified in the war years. With the start of World War I, she became concerned that sick and wounded soldiers should not be nursed by the unskilled, although many papers refused to publish Brodrick's call on this issue.[28] In 1915, she took on Lord Kitchener, the British Secretary of State for War, in public correspondence on the issue of the use of untrained nurses.

Brodrick and Irish Nationalism

However, political events in Ireland were now to have a marked effect on the development of Brodrick's thinking and her role in nursing. According to Maire Comerford, who witnessed the Easter Rising, joined Sinn Féin, and knew Brodrick from 1917 until her death, Brodrick was deeply affected by the rising and its aftermath. The woman who had already moved markedly from the background of her family by becoming a nurse and embracing the concerns of the poor in Kerry became an ardent Irish nationalist. Up until then, it was clear that she had not broken with her past completely. She had written poetry to mark the death of Queen Victoria[29] and even offered Ballincoona for members of the British Army injured in the war. Now, at fifty-five, her social and political ideals became even more radical, a radicalism that was to shape the remainder of her life and her approach to nursing politics. Her commitment to her new cause was expressed in her adoption of an Irish name: in the future, she often wrote in support of her new ideals as Gobnait Ni Bhruadair. She became a member of Cumann na mBan, the League of Women that supported the rising, and an ardent supporter of Sinn Féin, even becoming a Sinn Féin councillor in Kerry in 1920.[30] However, her support for Irish nationalist politics did not distract her from nursing politics and activities, which were also to become more radical.

Brodrick continued her support for the campaign for state registration. The College of Nursing, established in London in 1916, set up a Dublin Committee and then an Irish Board. However, this board was opposed by the Irish Nurses Association, of which Brodrick was a member, because it was a scheme for voluntary rather than statutory registration. Brodrick publicly denounced the Irish Board, from the position of both a supporter of state registration and an Irish nationalist.[31] The opponents of the College of Nursing Board's activities in Ireland then went on to form their own Irish Nursing Board, with an executive body that included Brodrick and the lady superintendents of the majority of Dublin hospitals.[32] This board was established to examine, certificate, and register nurses. Brodrick continued to attack against the development of the Irish Board of the College of Nursing, arguing, "The day is past when the medical profession can legislate for the sister profession of nursing. It is to our own profession alone that we owe allegiance, and by our own profession we intend to be governed."[33]

Brodrick spoke to nurses in Ireland and also to the National Union of Trained Nurses in England and the Scottish Nurses Association on the need for professional organization for nurses, the need for self-government, and the need for justice. What was required, she now argued, was "Fair pay for good work done, the limitation of working hours, such as every working woman was entitled to, recognition of their profession, and the acknowledgement of the services rendered to humanity by them."[34]

In the following years, Brodrick remained on the executive board of the Irish Nurses Association and continued to be re-elected to the Irish Nursing Board.[35] The ambitions of those supporting the campaign for state registration were realized with the passing of the Nurses Registration (Ireland) Act on December 23, 1919. However, in March, before this happened, Brodrick's commitment to the cause of nurse organization had led her to take a further step. Although the Irish Nurses Association did not support her initiative, Brodrick wrote to a meeting held at the Mansion House in support of the formation of a nurses' trade union to be allied with the Irish Women Workers' Union (IWWU).[36] The IWWU, established in 1911, was concerned with low-paid working-class women who were employed in appalling conditions. It had already been involved with the Lockout of 1913, when thousands of workers in Dublin were locked out from their jobs for seven months as employers tried not to recognize trade unions. Many other industrial disputes followed.

The association of the IWWU with industrial action and its membership of printers, laundresses, and textile factory workers were far from the image most nursing leaders were pursuing. The *Irish Times* expressed their sentiments when it asked nurses "not to dethrone and degrade the profession by dallying with the promises of Trade Unionism."[37] It is perhaps not surprising then that Brodrick was the only one of the prominent nurse leaders of the period in Ireland to support the creation of a trade union for nurses. In her call for members, she wrote, "It is full time that we nurses should awake out of sleep and take our rightful places amongst the workers of the world in fraternal organisation."[38] Now, she argued, although the Irish Nurses Association and the Irish Nursing Board had done well, a trade union was what was needed; what was required was a "fighting" body.[39] The Irish Nurses and Midwives Union was the result; its stated aim was "better salaries, shorter hours, less night duty, more freedom and control of their own profession."[40] It was opposed by all the other Irish nursing organizations of the day.

The other organizations, such as the Irish Nurses Association, were willing to acknowledge that these aims were "desirable objectives" but were opposed to a trade union as a means of gaining them. Still fighting for registration and professional recognition, they did not want to regard trained nurses as "workers" and implied that unionization would bring strike activity; "sound trade union lines" could never be applied to the position and role of nurses as they saw them.[41]

The position of the nursing associations and the other nursing leaders in opposing unionization in Ireland was reinforced by the strong belief in nursing as a vocation. This was not an attitude unique to Ireland, but it was reinforced there by the increasing role of religious orders in hospital work. Although the initial introduction of nurse training had been undertaken by Protestant bodies and in voluntary hospitals,[42] Catholic religious orders had established, controlled, and staffed new hospitals in the course of the nineteenth century and, at the end of the century, had also introduced training of Catholic lay nurses. The strong vocational nature of their work and approach had an impact on the way nursing was publicly regarded in Ireland.[43]

The union went ahead, however, and was established as a subsection of the IWWU. Although it kept Brodrick's support,[44] the union was not without problems in its first decade. These were mainly of a financial nature as it struggled to keep afloat and attract members, with concern expressed on occasion by its parent body, the IWWU, as to its likely viability.[45] However, it was this union and not the other nurses' organizations that survived, eventually evolving into the Irish Nurses Organisation, which today represents more than 31,000 nurses. Brodrick remained a committed member of the union for the rest of her life, being for some years Honorary Branch Secretary for Kerry. Even at her death in 1955, it was commented that it was only a few years earlier (i.e., in her eighties) that she had given up visiting the organization's headquarters in Dublin regularly.[46]

At a more local level, Brodrick's role as a nurse became intricately entwined with her politics as an Irish republican. During the civil war in Ireland, she took an active role in support of the republican men fighting against the treaty, and she is known to have hidden both men and arms during this period. She made no secret of her republican affiliations, and in May 1923, she was shot by government protreaty forces in Kerry when she refused to stop while cycling on a republican errand. From Kerry, she was transported to Dublin and imprisoned with the other female republican prisoners in the North Dublin Union. Now in her sixties, she immediately went on a hunger strike, despite her wounds. She wore her "well known blue nurses uniform" throughout her ordeal, and it was not until the fourteenth day of her hunger strike, when death seemed near, that she was released, having accepted that if she died this would in itself be worthwhile.

In her comments at the time, she illustrated her awareness of the impact of her birth and title. She had used them in the past to try to gain financial support for her hospital and cooperative, and now she reflected on their likely impact again, despite the fact that she reviled all that such titles stood for. "An old woman," she said, "is not much loss, but my death will be sure to make a noise, because of that wretched little prefix to my name, and in that way my death may do more good for Ireland than my life could do." And her eyes sparkled.[47]

Brodrick's republican sympathies ran hand in hand with her nursing commitment for the rest of her life. Even in the 1930s, visitors reported that she remained "dressed in the costume of a Princess Christian nurse."[48] The combination of the two, her republicanism and her nursing concern for the poor of rural Kerry, left her living in poverty, selling eggs in order to buy tea. She pressed republican literature on visitors and distributed it in local towns. One commentator, who met her when a boy, described how she "said [to him] to remember she had worn the same pair of boots for seventeen years."[49] In 1927, she gave a eulogy at the funeral of a fellow member of Cumann na mBan; the words she spoke then apply just as aptly to her own life: "Difficulties she faced squarely, looking straight through them. . . . The lesson that we learn from her life is a clear one. No compromise."[50]

"No Compromise"

It is clear that in Brodrick's contribution to nursing politics in Ireland that "no compromise" was her position to the end. In her life as a nurse, her social position, which she came to despise with her adoption of Irish Nationalist politics, brought her to the forefront of nursing in Britain and Ireland in the early twentieth century. However, she used this prominence in pursuit of the most critical goals for nurses at that period: state registration and professional organization. Alongside this, she became an outspoken speaker and advocate on one of the most controversial topics of the day, venereal disease. She followed her beliefs boldly and with confidence, even when this meant breaking with her family background through her support for Irish republicanism and opposing the other Irish nursing leaders, with whom she had worked so closely, with her continued support for a trade union rather than a mere professional organization for nurses. Born to the aristocracy, she finished her life in poverty but to her this was little import when her commitment and interventions helped bring to fruition the ideals she had for nurses.

ANN WICKHAM, BA, CERTED, MED, MSC, PHD
BNS Co-ordinator
Oscail
Dublin City University
Glasnevin
Dublin 9
Ireland

Acknowledgments

I want to thank the staff of the Department of Early Printed Books, Trinity College Library, University of Dublin, and Mr. E. Browne of the Local Studies and Archive Section, Kerry County Library, for their assistance.

Notes

1. In the period up until 1904, Brodrick is listed in *The Times* Court Circular as having attended many of the drawing rooms, state concerts, state balls, and garden parties held by the Queen at Buckingham Palace. She is also noted at other events held by senior

figures in the British establishment such as the archbishop of Canterbury. After 1904, the date of her departure for Ireland, Brodrick is absent from the Court Circular, except for her visit to the United States in 1912. All other mentions of her in *The Times* are in the news section and relate to her fund-raising for Ballincoona or to her republican activities. There is a gap in notices between 1901 and 1904, which may be accounted for by her period of training as a nurse, as she was qualified by 1904.

2. *Kerryman*, January 2, 1965, 7.

3. T.E. Stoakley, *Sneem: The Knot in the Ring* (Sneem: Sneem Tourism Association, 1986).

4. *British Journal of Nursing* (hereafter *BJN*), October 19, 1907, 310; *BJN*, April 10, 1909, 289: "For six weeks at a stretch I have been on duty eighteen hours daily, snatching my meals as best I could, and being called up at night as well."

5. *BJN*, July 24, 1909, 78.

6. The Congested Districts Board (CDB) was established by the British government in 1891 to promote economic and social development that could help alleviate the extreme poverty of the "congested" areas of the northwest, west, and southwest of Ireland, regarded as "overpopulated" in the sense that there was not an economic structure that could support the number of people in an area. The aim of the CDB was to replace erratic and inadequate charitable activities by sustainable development. CDB districts were also areas of high emigration as those unable to make a living in Ireland sought a future abroad.

7. *BJN*, August 6, 1910, 115.

8. *Kerryman*, January 2, 1965, 7.

9. *BJN*, May 6, 1911, 352.

10. *BJN*, September 9, 1911, 213.

11. *BJN*, September 28, 1912, 255.

12. *BJN*, August 16, 1913, 138; December 28, 1912, 517. Lavinia L. Dock and Mary Adelaide Nutting were the authors of *A History of Nursing: The Evolution of Nursing Systems from the Earliest Times to the Founding of the First English and American Training Schools for Nurses*, 4 vols. (London: Putnam, 1907–12). Dock, a high-profile American nursing leader, was, among other things, secretary of the American Federation of Nurses and of the International Council of Nurses and Honorary Member of the Matrons' Council of Great Britain and Ireland and of the German Nurses' Association.

13. *BJN*, August 16, 1913, 138; *BJN*, September 5, 1914, 195. The cost was more than £700,000 in today's values; www.eh.net/hmit/ukcompare

14. *BJN*, August 7, 1915, 109.

15. *BJN*, October 19, 1907, 310.

16. *BJN*, April 18, 1908, 311.

17. *BJN*, July 10, 1909, 21.

18. *BJN*, February 27, 1915, 177; *BJN*, June 1933.

19. The Honorable Sydney Holland (1855–1931), Chair of Poplar Hospital, London, from 1891 and Chairman of the London House Hospital Committee in 1896–1931, inherited the title Viscount Knutsford in 1914. He was a consistent opponent of state registration, arguing that the emphasis on examination would diminish the supply of nurses by excluding working-class women and fearing that registration would make nurses regard themselves as more superior than they should be in relation to the medical profession. See Brian Abel-Smith, *A History of the Nursing Profession* (London: Heinemann, 1960).

20. *BJN*, July 24, 1909, 78.

21. *BJN*, September 1937, 255.

22. *BJN*, October 30, 1909, 368.

23. The late nineteenth-century response to venereal disease had been to police prostitutes in an attempt to regulate the disease. Such a regulatory response was common at a European level and changed at different times in different countries. In Britain, the Contagious Diseases Acts promulgated in the 1860s and finally repealed in 1886 had allowed women to be arrested and examined and often forcibly confined in "Lock" hospitals. Brodrick's call predates the Royal Commission on VD in 1913, which is regarded as bringing a "new openness" to the topic, and which in 1916 was to promote a voluntary confidential clinic system as a more appropriate response. See Roger Davidson and Lesley A. Hall, *Sex, Sin and Suffering: Venereal Disease and European Society Since 1870* (London: Routledge, 2001); Lesley A. Hall, "*The Great Scourge": Syphilis as a Medical Problem and Moral Metaphor, 1880–1916* (1998), homepages.primex.co.uk/~lesleyah/grtscrge.htm

24. She was to claim she was "everything in turn from a maid of all work to a doctor, including housekeeper, farmhand, head quarryman, plasterer, contractor, nurse and president of a co-operative society." *BJN*, May 6, 1911, 352. Her concern for the health of children was not confined to venereal disease and its impact; in a major denunciation of the upper levels of society, she also attacked attempts at contraception and abortion. *BJN*, April 22, 1911, 323.

25. *BJN*, May 31, 1913, 430. The recognition of her eminence in the nursing profession in Ireland can be seen from her place in the reception given to mark the start of the conference. "The procession was in the following order: Mrs. Bedford Fenwick and Miss Huxley (President of the INA), Lady Hermione Blackwood and Miss Ramsden, the Hon. Albinia Brodrick and Miss Cunningham." *BJN*, June 14, 1913, 482.

26. *BJN*, January 13, 1912. The United Irishwomen was established in 1910 by a group of middle-class women inspired by the work of George Russell and the Irish Agricultural organization. They aimed to improve the life of rural women for the good of the country, with an emphasis on self-help and cooperation. The deficiency of health care in rural areas was an early concern, especially the lack of nurses for the rural poor. The provision of nurses in rural areas became one of the primary aims of the organization. See Aileen Heverin, *The Irish Countrywomen's Association: A History* (Dublin: Wolfhound, 2000).

27. The nurse in question, Margaret Cowman, was only trained for seven months at Charing Cross Hospital when sent there by the United Irishwomen. However, she attended the Rotunda in Dublin for refresher courses every two years and remained in the post from 1912 to 1963. *Irish Medical Journal*, 94, no. 7 (July/August 2001); *BJN*, June 21, 1913, 507.

28. *BJN*, November 21, 1914, 412; *BJN*, January 9, 1915, 32; *BJN*, April 3, 1915, 281.

29. Included in Albinia Brodrick, *Verses of Adversity* (London: Henry Froude, 1904).

30. Cumann na mBan, the League of Women, was formed in 1914 as an auxiliary corps to complement the Irish Volunteer Force (IVF), which had been launched as a paramilitary body in 1913 and comprised the majority of those who took part in the Easter Rising. Cumann na mBan's recruits were mainly white-collar workers and professional women, but a significant proportion were from the working class. Although it was otherwise an independent organization, its executive was subordinate to that of the volunteers. After the rising, Cumann na mBan, led by Countess Markievicz, organized prisoner relief agencies

and canvassed for Sinn Féin in the 1918 general election. During the Anglo-Irish war, its members hid arms and provided safe houses for volunteers. Most of its members opposed the treaty. Sinn Féin was established as a political party in 1905, with a policy that declared that the Act of Union of Great Britain and Ireland was illegal. At first it attracted minimal support. However, Sinn Féin was wrongly blamed by the British for the Easter Rising, with which it then had little association. Then surviving leaders of the rising, under Éamon de Valera, took over the party. Support was subsequently boosted by the public anger over the execution of rising leaders. In the general election of December 1918, Sinn Féin won 73 of Ireland's 106 seats in the United Kingdom parliament. In January 1919, Sinn Féin MPs assembled in Dublin's Mansion House and proclaimed themselves the Parliament of Ireland, Dáil Éireann. Sinn Féin subsequently underwent successive splits (1922, 1926, 1970, and 1986), from which other parties developed.

31. *BJN*, February 24, 1917, 137.

32. *BJN*, May 26, 1917, 365.

33. *BJN*, October 6, 1917, 221.

34. *BJN*, December 1, 1917, 354.

35. *BJN*, March 23, 1918, 208; *BJN*, July 13, 1918.

36. *BJN*, March 8, 1919, 156.

37. *Irish Times*, February 28, 1919, quoted in R. Cullen Owens, *A Social History of Women in Ireland* (Dublin: Gill and Macmillan, 2005), 200.

38. *BJN*, March 29, 1919, 207.

39. *BJN*, March 22, 1919, 192.

40. *BJN*, March 8, 1919, 158.

41. *BJN*, March 8, 1919, 158.

42. Ann Wickham, "A Better Scheme for Nursing: The Influence of the Dublin Hospital Sunday Fund on Nursing and Nurse Training in the Nineteenth Century," *International History of Nursing Journal*, 6, no. 2 (2001): 26–35.

43. For articles exploring this impact, see Maria Luddy, "Nuns as Workhouse Nurses, 1861–1898," in *Medicine, Disease and the State in Ireland*, 1650–1940, ed. Elizabeth Malcolm and Greta Jones (Cork: Cork University Press, 1999), 102–20; M.Ó. hÓgartaigh, "Flower Power and 'Mental Grooviness': Nurses and Midwives in Ireland in the Early Twentieth Century," in *Women and Paid Work in Ireland, 1500–1930*, ed. Bernadette Whelan (Dublin: Four Courts Press, 2000), 133–47.

44. *BJN*, January 14, 1922.

45. Irish Women Workers Union, Executive Minutes 1919–1931, Irish Museum of Labour History.

46. *Irish Nurses Magazine*, February 1955, 9.

47. Margaret Buckley, *The Jangle of the Keys* (Dublin: Duffy, 1938), 64.

48. Tilly Fleischmann, *Some Reminiscences of Arnold Bax* (1955), http://|www.musicweb.uk.net/|bax/|Tilly3.htm

49. *Kerryman*, January 2, 1965, 7.

50. *Saoirse–Irish Freedom* 7, 7 (n.d.).

"The Ultimate Destination of All Nursing": The Development of District Nursing in England, 1880–1925

CARRIE HOWSE
University of Gloucestershire

Florence Nightingale is chiefly remembered for the reform of hospital nursing in the late nineteenth century, but scant attention has been paid to her involvement in the establishment and development of district nursing throughout England. Nightingale believed that the future of nursing lay in district nursing, with its dual aims of curative care and preventive education, yet historians of British nursing tend to concentrate on general nursing in the hospital setting because that is where training occurred.[1] District nursing, if it is mentioned at all in such studies, is seen as only a footnote to the broader context of social history and philanthropy. The only official histories of district nursing were written by Mary Stocks and Monica Baly in 1960 and 1987, respectively,[2] and these two slim volumes remain the main sources on Queen Victoria's Jubilee Institute for Nurses (QVJI), the central body that standardized training and unified existing philanthropic schemes through its system of affiliation and inspection. Baly uses Stocks as her main secondary source, and although both books are factual and informative, their scope is limited by the fact that they were commissioned to celebrate milestones in the history of district nursing. They are, therefore, designed to be congratulatory and to emphasize positive progress over the years. They concentrate on the leading figures of the movement, not on the nurses themselves, and on details of politics and administration, not on the day-to-day duties and problems involved in nursing the sick poor in their own homes.

It is the aim of this article to help redress this imbalance in the historiography of nursing. By examining Nightingale's views and aims, I argue that the organizational structure of QVJI came closest of all branches of the profession to her vision of the future of nursing. The extent to which her theories were achieved in practice will be considered through the analysis of the Queen's Roll, which records the personal and career details of each Queen's nurse. In particular, I will show how the difficulties experienced in recruiting

Nursing History Review 15 (2007): 65–94. A publication of the American Association for the History of Nursing. Copyright © 2007 Springer Publishing Company.

nurses for rural districts led to the introduction of a second grade of district nurse, the Village Nurse-Midwives. By analyzing the records of District Nursing Associations in Gloucestershire, where the rural branch of QVJI was founded, I discuss why QVJI failed to attract the class of recruits Nightingale envisaged and how, nevertheless, it became central to national health and welfare policies.

The Metropolitan Nursing Association

By the 1880s, the Nightingale reforms had clearly had an effect on hospital nursing in England, despite the entrenched views and professional jealousy of some doctors. The infirmary wards of workhouses had also been reformed and improved, and in rural areas almost 300 cottage hospitals had been established, which provided respite care for four to ten patients with a trained resident nurse and regular visits by a general practitioner.

However, Nightingale herself believed that "the ultimate destination of all nursing is the nursing of the sick in their own homes."[3] As early as 1866, she had "resolved to give herself to District Nursing."[4] At that time, Nightingale was offering advice and support to William Rathbone, a philanthropic merchant who was establishing a scheme of district nursing in his home town of Liverpool. At Nightingale's suggestion, in 1862, the Liverpool Training School and Home for Nurses was opened in connection with the Liverpool Royal Infirmary. Thus, the precedent was set that district nurses should be hospital trained, preferably under the Nightingale reformed system, as well as being specially trained in district work. By 1867, the city of Liverpool had been divided into eighteen districts, each with its own nurses.

In 1868, Rathbone was elected a Liberal MP and consequently spent part of each year in London. The personal contact this enabled him to make with Nightingale led to a lifelong friendship and mutual admiration. When, in 1874, Sir Edward Lechmere of the English branch of the Order of St. John of Jerusalem proposed that a system of district nursing should be set up in London, Rathbone and Nightingale were asked to help. Nightingale was at that time at the family home in Derbyshire. Her father had died in January, and she had temporarily returned to care for her mother, who was eighty-six, frail, and confused. Nightingale was therefore unable to personally organize the London scheme, but, as with the Liverpool system, she did everything that could be done from a distance. In 1874, she wrote a pamphlet, *Suggestions for Improving the Nursing Service for the Sick Poor*, and she recommended that a detailed survey be carried out on the district nursing needs and existing provision in London. For this task, she selected Florence Lees (later Mrs. Dacre Craven), an experienced nurse who had trained at the Nightingale School at St. Thomas' Hospital. Lees's survey covered twenty-two organizations, mainly religious and philanthropic bodies, which among them provided only 106 district nurses for the whole of London. Many of these nurses were only partially or barely trained at all; in the case of the Ranyard Bible Nurses, their original aim was to teach the Christian religion to the poor.

Mary Stocks describes Lees's subsequent report as one of the most important social surveys of the Victorian age,[5] and as a result of her findings, the Metropolitan Nursing Association (MNA) was formed in 1875. The Duke of Westminster accepted the chairmanship and Lees was appointed superintendent general, responsible for recruiting and overseeing the trainees, who, after completing the standard one year's training as Lady Probationers at the Nightingale School, were to be trained specifically as district nurses. The MNA was based at 23 Bloomsbury Square, which provided an office for Lees and comfortable accommodations for five nurses. The first MNA trainees worked an eight-hour day, six hours in their district with the other two hours devoted to lectures or reading. They were allowed two hours leisure time in the evening and were guaranteed eight hours sleep a night. This rigorous training, which combined personal devotion with technical excellence, reflected Nightingale's belief that, to fulfill the grueling and responsible duties involved in caring for the sick poor in their own homes, "a district nurse . . . must be of a yet higher class and of a yet fuller training than a hospital nurse, because she has not the doctor always at hand; because she has no hospital appliances at hand at all; and because she has to take notes of the case for the doctor, who has no one but her to report to him. She is his staff of clinical clerks, dressers, and nurses."[6]

In response, *The Lancet* expressed the opinion that district nurses would be better employed by "the class who have some education, but who for the most part perform their own domestic work and keep no servants," such as clerks and warehousemen, for whom "the acceptance of help should not involve any loss of self-respect."[7]

The Lancet also dismissed Nightingale's definition of the purpose of district nursing, which she envisaged as the dual aims of curative care and preventive education: "Now, what is a district nurse to do? A nurse is, first, to nurse. Secondly, to nurse the room as well as the patient – to put the room into nursing order; that is, to make the room such as a patient can recover in; to bring care and cleanliness into it, and to teach the inmates to keep up that care and cleanliness. Thirdly, to bring such sanitary defects as produce sickness and death . . . to the notice of the public officer whom it concerns."[8]

In *The Lancet*'s view, such an approach would only cause further problems, as the poor "resent the intrusion of strangers" and if "a district nurse spies out the filthiness of a home, and makes a report which brings down inspectors . . . [she] is likely to become a most unpopular personage."[9]

Nightingale also believed that the district nurse must look for the means of mitigating suffering, even in incurable cases, and teach by example,

> to sweep and dust away, to empty and wash out all the appalling dirt and foulness; to air and disinfect; rub the windows, sweep the fireplace, carry out and shake the bits of old sacking and carpet, and lay them down again; fetch fresh water and fill the kettle; wash the patient and the children, and make the bed. . . . And it requires a far higher stamp of woman . . . thus to combine the servant with the teacher, and with the gentlewoman, . . . [and] command the patient's confidence . . . than almost any other work.[10]

The Lancet countered by questioning the efficacy of encouraging the poor to remain in "unwholesome dwellings" during sickness when they could be removed to a hospital. They suggested that the £20,000 that Nightingale hoped to raise for the MNA would be better spent building "a hospital of one hundred beds" or improved housing for the poor than providing "women who, in spite of training and an ability to take temperatures and scientific notes, might not always be a welcome addition to a small household."[11]

However, *The Lancet* had always been critical of Nightingale's theories, particularly her belief that nurses should be educated ladies who could influence the behavior of the working classes through the power of social example as well as caring for them. The very purpose of district nursing, in Nightingale's opinion, was to separate the sick poor from each other rather than grouping them together in hospitals, and it appears that the public, the media, and the majority of the medical profession in London did not support *The Lancet*'s contrary view. When Nightingale's letter to *The Times* was reprinted as a pamphlet, *On Trained Nursing for the Sick Poor*, it ran to two editions, and doctors in working-class areas acknowledged the value of the nurses' services.

The last quarter of the nineteenth century was in general a period of political and social reform. A plethora of wide-ranging legislation was passed in response to the growing awareness that the material conditions of the poor were as essential a part of paternalism as salvation of the soul. This combination of social and religious motives was manifest in the growing numbers and variety of urban visiting societies, whose volunteers could be found in hospitals, workhouses, prisons, and asylums, as well as in the homes of the poor. As social historian Frank Prochaska expresses it, "Armed with the paraphernalia of their calling – Bibles, tracts, blankets, food and coal tickets, and love – these foot-soldiers of the charitable army went from door to door to combat the evils of poverty, disease, and irreligion. In other words, they sought to reform family life through a moral and physical cleansing of the nation's homes."[12]

Furthermore, the replacement of the Poor Law Board by the Local Government Board under the Act of 1871 brought public health into the same administrative department as poor relief. The subsequent series of acts during the 1870s, which consolidated previous attempts at sanitary reform, also saw the appointment of medical officers of health responsible for effecting national policies at the local level. This was a clear indication that the state should accept responsibility for the health of the people, including provision for the sick poor. In this context of national reform, the establishment and success of the MNA can be seen as reflecting the recognized need to improve the lives of the poor. Its work was confined to London, but Nightingale predicted that "within a few years . . . [it] will be a disgrace . . . to any district . . . not to have a good District Nurse to nurse the sick poor at home."[13] The opportunity to translate her vision into reality came in 1887.

Queen Victoria's Jubilee Institute for Nurses

In that year, Queen Victoria celebrated her Golden Jubilee and the women of England were invited to make donations to a Jubilee Fund. Three million women subscribed a total of £82,000 and, after personal gifts of jewelry had been designed and executed by Carringtons of Regent Street and a statue of Prince Albert commissioned for Windsor Park, suggestions were invited for how the remaining £70,000 should be spent.

Florence Nightingale and her supporters saw the opportunity not only to place the MNA on a solid financial footing but also to extend its work throughout England. William Rathbone prepared a draft plan, which was then sent to Nightingale for her comments and input, particularly concerning the selection and training of district nurses. When the final plan was submitted for the Queen's consideration, it was chosen in preference to several other suggestions, such as supporting emigration. Queen Victoria was known to be sympathetic to nursing and she had followed Nightingale's career with interest. In addition, the Duke of Westminster, chairman of the MNA, was also chairman of the Jubilee Fund. These links were, without doubt, important in influencing the Queen's choice of how the Jubilee Fund should be spent, but Monica Baly believes that the establishment of a national district nursing scheme was also made possible by "the changing social scene, the new awareness of the health needs of the community, together with the greater emancipation and better education of women at the end of the century, [which] brought it within the bounds of possibility."[14]

On September 20, 1889, a Royal Charter was issued, formally establishing QVJI. The first Council of twenty-two members, selected by the Queen herself, included the Duke of Westminster, William Rathbone, Henry Bonham Carter, and the Reverend and Mrs. Craven (formerly Miss Lees), all of them known supporters of Nightingale and her methods. The degree of royal approval of and involvement in district nursing was further reflected by the inclusion on the Council of all three of Her Majesty's own daughters who were still resident in Britain at that time, Their Royal Highnesses the Princesses Christian, Louise, and Beatrice.

This Queen's Council accepted the MNA as the model for the new QVJI. Its training and syllabus were adopted, as was its most important and innovative precept, that its nurses should be supervised not by religious bodies or by philanthropic laity who knew little or nothing of nursing but by superintendents and inspectors who were themselves both educated ladies and highly trained nurses. Existing urban district nursing associations, which conformed to the general principles of the foundation, were invited to apply for affiliation with QVJI. One of the first was Rathbone's own scheme in Liverpool, whose pioneering work in the 1860s had now, he said, spread "far beyond anything that even the most sanguine of us could then foresee."[15]

Rural areas were brought into the scheme by the affiliation in 1892 and eventual amalgamation in 1897 of the Rural Nursing Association (RNA), a national charity that had been founded in Gloucestershire in 1890 by a free-thinking intellectual, Elizabeth Malleson, and the altruistic Lucy Hicks-Beach, Countess St. Aldwyn.[16] Small, independent rural nursing schemes set up by local philanthropic individuals already existed, but they were scattered all over England. As for their urban counterparts, the standard of their nurses' training varied, and some, such as the Cottage Benefit Nursing Association, founded by Miss Bertha Broadwood in 1883, provided nurses who lived in with their poor patients. The RNA was the first national rural district nursing organization, offering both nursing care and midwifery by trained visiting nurses, and by inviting existing isolated schemes to join, it established and maintained national standards of trained district nursing, controlled by a central body. By the time it was designated as QVJI's Rural District Branch, its nurses were working in twenty-five counties, and its impressive list of committee members and supporters included two duchesses, nine countesses, four viscountesses, and seventeen ladies. The organizational structure adopted by the RNA reflected the importance of the social hierarchy as it then existed, and it was incorporated into QVJI's own system when they amalgamated (see Figure 1).

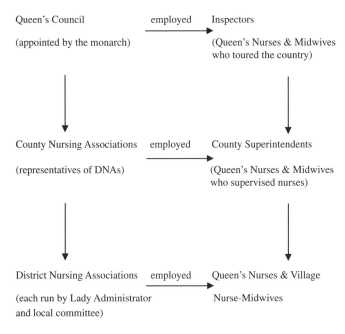

Figure 1. Organizational structure of QVJI.

At the local level, the manager of the District Nursing Association (DNA) was more often than not the local "Lady Bountiful," and the committee would consist of her daughters and worthy matrons such as the wives of the vicar, doctor, and headmaster. At the county level, the senior administrative posts of the County Nursing Association (CNA) would be filled by the ladies of the highest social rank and status; thus, in Gloucestershire, the county president was the Duchess of Beaufort and the vice president was the Countess St. Aldwyn. The county superintendent, who was herself under the supervision of QVJI inspectors, was to be a Queen's nurse (QN), and her appointment by the CNA required the approval of the Council of QVJI. The committee of each DNA was responsible for fund-raising, paying the nurse's salary, and providing suitable accommodation. In this way, the importance of the church and the social elite in rural areas was recognized and acknowledged; the prerogative and influence of the hierarchical society, with its accompanying overtones of noblesse oblige, remained operational; and the social fabric was not disturbed. At the same time, the quality of training, qualification, and subsequent day-to-day nursing was standardized on Nightingale lines by the requirement of annual reports from the DNAs and CNAs to the Council of QVJI and inspection of the nurses' work.

From its instigation, QVJI recommended that its nurses "should all be duly approved women of excellent personal character, and of good education."[17] In its comment on this announcement, *The Times* assumed that, "bearing in mind what are the highest attributes of feminine character," QVJI would "provide a congenial vocation for numbers of refined and good women, and enable them to indulge their tenderest instincts unclogged by pecuniary considerations.... And some of the atmosphere of refinement which may be expected to surround a Queen's nurse will stay in the house when the nurse's mission is ended and she is gone."[18] In a letter to the newspaper, an unidentified doctor stressed that it was "manifestly essential" that such representatives of "Her Majesty's benevolent desires" should be "in all respects worthy, . . . in good health, of good character, of assured sobriety"; the treasurer of the North London Nursing Association added that "this class of superior nurses" should be so "worthy and self-sacrificing" that the idea of "making broad her phylactery" would be "generally distasteful" to them.[19]

From these comments it can be seen that, despite the general agreement that the aim of district nurses should be to improve the lives of the poor and to care for them, there was a clear difference of opinion concerning motivation. On the one hand, the media and public were calling for a pseudoreligious order that reflected the belief that philanthropy was the highest expression of women's "natural" virtuous traits. On the other hand, Florence Nightingale envisaged paid professionals who were, nevertheless, inspired by a sense of calling. She believed that, as "man cannot live by bread alone . . . [so] woman does not live by wages alone."[20] She recognized the danger that district nursing could be seen by young women as the means "to have a life of freedom, with an interesting employment, for a few years – to do as little as you can and amuse yourself as much as you can," and she warned of the danger of district nurses responding to "fashion . . . [with] its consequent want of earnestness . . . [and] the enthusiasm which every one . . . must have in order to follow her calling properly."[21] She reiterated her definition of the purpose of district nursing by differentiating between nursing the sick ("to help the patient suffering from disease to live") and what she called "health-nursing" ("to keep or put the constitution of the healthy child or human being in such a state as to have no disease").[22]

By that time, Nightingale was also advocating the employment of health-missioners. These were to be educated ladies who were not nurses but who would be trained to give lectures and instruction to the poor on sanitation and hygiene. She acknowledged that such women might prove difficult to find in sparsely populated areas, and she stressed that in isolated rural communities the district nurse "also should be a health missioner as well as a sick-nurse." By acting as "missioners of health-at-home," district nurses had the opportunity to address firsthand the social evils of "dirt, drink, diet, damp, draughts, drains"; to achieve this, "the nurse must have method, self-sacrifice, watchful activity, love of the work, devotion to duty, . . . courage, . . . the tenderness of the mother, the absence of the prig . . . and never, never let the nurse forget that she must look for the fault of the nursing, as much as for the fault of the disease, in the symptoms of the patient."[23]

Nightingale's views were formally embodied in *A Guide to District Nurses and Home Nursing*, a manual Mrs. Craven was asked to write for the use of QVJI nurses in 1889, and which Nightingale proofread. Nightingale's influence is clear, particularly where Craven stresses that a district nurse must be motivated by "a real love for the poor, and a real desire to lessen the misery she may see among them. . . . Her aim must be not only to aid in curing disease and alleviating pain, but also through the illness of one member of a family to gain an influence for good so as to raise the whole family. . . . Wherever a district nurse enters, order and cleanliness should enter with her . . . [and] every poor person should be as well and as tenderly nursed as if he were the highest in the land."[24]

Training of Queen's Nurses

To achieve these high standards, QVJI required the following qualifications in 1890:

(a) Training at some approved general hospital or infirmary for not less than one year.
(b) Approved training in district nursing for not less than six months, including the nursing of mothers and their infants after childbirth.
(c) Nurses in country districts must have at least three months' approved training in midwifery.[25]

The distinction between clauses (b) and (c) was an important one. QNs working in towns were not expected to undertake midwifery cases, but they could attend to a mother and baby after birth if a doctor decided they needed nursing attention as opposed to routine postnatal care. QNs in rural areas were expected to be qualified for midwifery cases but only as a precautionary measure; it was stressed that "the duties of the midwife, as distinguished from a nurse, are not to be undertaken, except in cases of emergency." However, midwifery formed an important part of the RNA's work, and under the terms of its Constitution as the Rural District Branch, QVJI's Council compromised between what it considered desirable and what was practically possible in remote areas: "The services of the midwives are intended for those who cannot afford doctors' fees." Because this applied to the majority of poor rural families, midwifery was clearly established as an integral part of a rural district nurse's duties.

A Medical & Sanitary Subcommittee was formed, whose members included Craven, and the syllabus they devised ensured that the subjects not taught to nurses in hospitals figured prominently in the training of QNs. The syllabus reflected Nightingale's dual aims of curative care and preventive education by including sanitary reform, teaching health matters, ventilation, drainage, water supply, diets for the healthy and the sick, the feeding of infants, infectious diseases, monthly nursing of lying-in women, and the care of newborn infants. All these subjects had to be covered in the six months' training course, along with practical work, and were tested by a three-hour written examination in which six questions had to be answered.

The additional midwifery training was equally demanding. Under the Midwives Act of 1902, the widely recognized and accepted examination of the London Obstetrical Society was replaced by a similar examination conducted by the newly formed Central Midwives Board and held four times a year. The training period for midwives was set at only three months, and the examination was partly written and partly oral. The written examination, like the paper for QNs, consisted of six questions to be completed in three hours, while the oral examination was of fifteen minutes' duration.

Social historian Jane Lewis states that the initial training period was set so short for fear of creating a shortage, and that the midwives themselves pressed for a longer period of training, believing that it would improve their professional status and make the work more popular among "a superior class of women." In 1916, the training period for untrained women was doubled to six months, but it remained three months for trained nurses. This coincided with World War I and, consequently, a shortage of male doctors on the home front, many of them having volunteered for duty in the Army Medical Corps.

The resulting increase in births attended by midwives continued after 1918, particularly in rural districts, and reports on maternal mortality, produced by Dame Janet Campbell of the Ministry of Health in 1923 and 1927, "emphasised the particularly fine record of the QVJI midwives, who served all of England and Wales with the exception of Wiltshire, Essex and Northumberland, attending 80,147 cases (10%) in 1924. Where they worked . . . the maternal mortality rate was half the national rate."[26] This statistic does not differentiate between home deliveries by a midwife alone and difficult cases where a doctor was called in to assist. However, the thorough and demanding training of QVJI nurses ensured that they recognized such difficult cases and knew when to send for medical assistance, which fact alone could be instrumental in saving both mother and child.

In 1924, the training period for midwives was again doubled, to twelve months for untrained women and six months for trained nurses. Meanwhile, QVJI's district training course for QNs remained at its original six months, while the prior qualification of not less than one year's experience in a general hospital or infirmary in 1890 was increased in 1906 to "not less than three years' training in approved hospitals or infirmaries."[27] Thus, QVJI specified a uniform length of training and standard of qualifications for all its nurses starting in 1890, twelve years before the Midwives Act and almost thirty years before the introduction of the Registration Act. In fact, the Queen's Roll was established at the very time that Florence Nightingale was battling with the Royal British Nurses' Association (RBNA) over the attempt of the latter to provide a register of qualified nurses.

Founded and led by the formidable Mrs. Ethel Bedwick Fenwick, who had been made Matron of St. Bartholomew's Hospital, London, at the age of twenty-four, the RBNA was agitating for a standard certificate of proficiency that would be awarded by an independent body of examiners rather than by the individual hospital at which a nurse had trained. The nurse would then be entitled to have her name placed on a national register of nurses. Nightingale believed that, even after thirty years of reform, nursing was still too unorganized and divergent for an official national register, and she used her considerable influence to ensure the charter granted to the RBNA in 1893 omitted the word "register" and conferred only the right to the "maintenance of a list of persons who may have applied to have their names entered thereon as nurses."[28] In her definitive biography, Cecil Woodham-Smith stresses that Nightingale

> was not necessarily against registration, but she was passionately opposed to the kind of registration proposed. The qualifying of a nurse by examination only took no account of the character training which she held to be as important as the acquisition of technical skill.... Nor in her opinion would the register as proposed protect the public. The fact that a nurse's name was on it would only mean that at a certain date she had satisfied the examiners in certain tests; it would tell nothing of her subsequent record. If a register were to be useful it should be kept up to date, and include a description of each nurse's character.[29]

Such a scheme was never achieved for general nurses, but from its inception, QVJI, with its national system of supervision and regular inspections, did ensure that, once qualified, its nurses continued to maintain standards, and its centrally held records provided exactly the type of comments that Nightingale deemed essential, covering character and conduct as well as work. The Queen's Roll records the personal and career details of each QN, including date of birth, marital status, religious denomination, education, father's occupation, own previous occupation, hospital training and nursing experience, district training, certificates and badges, and reports on posts held. These unique records offer a fascinating insight into the lives of the QNs, and also offer the opportunity to consider the extent to which QVJI's aims were met in practice.

The Queen's Roll

As we have seen, Florence Nightingale believed that, to fulfill her dual aims of curative care and preventive education, a district nurse needed to be an educated lady. Craven boasted that some of the earliest applicants to train with the MNA had been presented at court as debutantes. However, surviving records of paternal occupations among the 539 nurses listed on the Queen's Roll in 1896 include several clergymen, an Oxford professor, a solicitor, a bank manager, two army officers, and a farmer, which suggests a predominantly middle-class background. Among the earliest QNs, Alpha Fenton, who qualified in 1892, was the daughter of an auctioneer and listed her own previous occupation as "housekeeper to brothers." The records of Leah Garratt, who qualified in 1890, do not include her father's occupation, but Leah remained "at home" until she began her hospital training at Worcester in 1886 at the age of twenty-one, which, again, suggests a comfortable background.[30]

This trend continued in the early years of the twentieth century. Of a sample of twelve nurses who qualified as QNs between 1902 and 1908, only two (17 percent) record a previous occupation: Alexina Cowee and Ann Newdick, both of whom had been children's nurses and were the daughters of farmers. The other ten (83 percent) either give no previous occupation or are listed as "at home." Where father's occupation is recorded, these include a printer, a merchant, and two clergymen. The father of Olive Goddard was "in Her Late Majesty's consular service in China," while Margaret Powell, daughter of an army officer, was recorded as being "refined and nice in her ideas though not a lady by birth."[31]

By 1913, one of the items for discussion at a Conference of Superintendents was, "It seems that the type of woman now taking up district work is not what it used to be, judging from those applying. . . . Can anything be done to make this work more attractive to the woman wishing to devote herself to work amongst the sick poor?"[32] Any points raised or conclusions reached were not recorded, but, among QNs who qualified between 1910 and 1917, 43 percent had worked prior to hospital training, their occupations including a cashier and a flosser. Paternal occupations included an engineer, two bootmakers, a florist, and a grocer, which suggests a more upper working-class than lower middle-class background.[33]

When the question of the nurses' social background was discussed again in 1922, it was "thought that nurses did not apply as they formerly did because there were now many more professions open to women, district work was hard, the nurses objected to further training after the three years in hospital, . . . the thought of another examination and the binding of a year's agreement were deterrents, as also was the knowledge that there was no pension after the term of service."[34]

Among QNs who qualified between 1919 and 1925, paternal occupations now included two engineers, a postman, and a master joiner, and 67 percent of the nurses had previously worked, their occupations including shop assistants and a clerk. Social background alone is, of course, no definite indicator of intelligence and practical nursing ability. Susie Bayliss, a former serving maid, was described as "a most capable, practical nurse," and she rose to become assistant superintendent in Portsmouth from 1930 to 1937.[35]

All candidates for training as QNs had to have already qualified as hospital nurses, although before the Registration Act, the length and quality of their training varied. Nevertheless, the requirement of this prior qualification, together with the breadth and depth of technical and theoretical knowledge demanded by the district training, assumed a certain level of ability and literacy. In fact, the Queen's Roll suggests that some candidates struggled to achieve the required standard. The examination paper for QNs carried sixty marks, and although the minimum pass mark and pass rate are not known, where examination results are recorded, comments on marks below 75 percent cite educational difficulties, particularly for working-class candidates (see Table 1). Beatrice Price, a grocer's daughter, was noted throughout her career to be "not a good record keeper" whose "ante-natal records suggest paperwork is rather difficult."[36]

Once qualified, a QN would be sent for one year to a post arranged by QVJI, after which she was free to apply for a vacancy of her choice. In towns, a central home was provided because Nightingale believed that the morale, health, and reputation of the district nurses would suffer if they did not enjoy the same safe respectability and warm supportive companionship that her vision of the ideal hospital nurses' home would provide. However, in many hospitals, as feminist historian Martha Vicinus expresses it, "descriptions of life in the nurses' home sound like a combination of boot camp and boarding school . . . with stringent and often unnecessary regulations enforced by ancient and unrelenting battle-axes. . . . Meals were remembered as dreary and hasty affairs, without relaxation of discipline. . . . The elaborate system of times off and on made it difficult to

Table 1.   Results of the Examination for the Roll of Queen's Nurses

Year	Nurse's surname	Mark out of 60	Percent	Comments
1908	Newdick	42	70	Many parts good considering apparent educational difficulty
1908	Sproat	46	76.7	Not very energetic
1910	Lee	47	78	Some parts very good
1910	Milford	54	90	Very good
1911	Douglas	39½	65.8	Question 3 surprisingly poorly answered by this candidate
1911	Tatton	41½	69	Some parts fairly good, limited abilities
1911	Griffiths	44½	74	A good nurse but lacks finish
1912	Paling	35	58	Handicapped by limited abilities and education
1917	Price	38	63	Scanty, too sketchy
1919	Boston	49	81.7	Not good at clerical work
1923	Jenkins	51	85	Nervous and excitable
1924	Webb, F.M.	34½	57.5	Is not very well educated
1924	Webb, L.F.	33½	55.8	Lacking in education
1924	Avery	45½	75.8	Very capable and methodical

Source: CMAC SA/QNI/J.3.

keep the dining room clean and the food fresh. . . . Little variety and much starch depressed everyone."[37]

It is perhaps not difficult to imagine that an urban district nurses' home, located within the community the nurses served, with fewer staff than a hospital, would have created a more homelike, intimate, and supportive atmosphere. At Stroud in Gloucestershire, three nurses took up residence at "The Home" in 1895, under the superintendence of a Miss Blackwell. By 1898, their number had increased to six, and patients were attended not only in Stroud itself but also in nine surrounding villages. The Annual Reports of the Stroud DNA regularly acknowledge gifts of flowers, fruit, and vegetables that had been "gratefully received at the Nurses' Home," which suggests a cheerful ambience and healthy diet.[38] Similarly, between fifteen and twenty nurses shared the Victoria Home in Cheltenham from 1905 to 1925, and thanks were regularly expressed "to Mr Beadnell, who tunes the piano without charge," to "Messrs Webb Bros [who] have very generously supplied the Home with firewood, free of cost," and to "Messrs Jack & Co [who] attend to the hall clock free of charge."[39] The house was supplied with a hot-water system for which "the pipes were passed through a large cupboard, and this gives a place for drying the nurses' cloaks in wet weather," while "a well-built weather-proof house in the garden" was installed "which could accommodate sixteen bicycles." QVJI Inspectors concluded that "the Home was comfortable, the food was excellent and abundant … and, though hard work is done, the Staff and the pupils are happy." When Caroline Coaling was superintendent of the nurses' home in Southampton from 1910 to 1921, she was reported to be "an excellent housekeeper [who] makes her nurses happy and comfortable."[40] By 1922, it was reported that "in England and Wales there were 17 Homes with staffs above 10 nurses, 123 with staffs of from 4 to 10, 49 with staffs of 3 [and] 152 Districts with 2 nurses."[41]

Such communal arrangements were only possible in urban areas, and in rural areas the majority of district nurses lived alone. They were provided either with board and lodging in two furnished rooms, with attendance, fuel, and light, or with a rented cottage. Although some nurses enjoyed the independence, responsibility, and sense of achievement such a post could offer, others found that they had exchanged a restrictive hospital life for one of isolation, and in 1922, the *Queen's Nurses' Magazine* noted that "the loneliness of a single district was very trying."[42]

Whether employed in an urban or a rural district, each nurse worked alone, and it is clear from the records that many were conscious of the importance of their role in the community. Although the certificate of the London Obstetrical Society (LOS) was still recognized and its possession automatically admitted a nurse to the new Roll of Midwives opened by the Central Midwives Board (CMB) in October 1903, some of the earliest QNs also took the new examination. Alpha Fenton, who had passed the LOS Certificate in 1892, also gained the CMB Certificate in 1904. Similarly, Fanny Mellor, who passed the LOS Certificate in February 1903, only eight months before the Midwives Roll opened, took the CMB Certificate a year later, while Helen Moore passed the LOS Certificate in July 1903 and took the CMB Certificate just six months later.[43] The fact that an additional certificate was not compulsory for these nurses, who were already practicing QNs, suggests that they were anxious to be seen as up-to-date professionals.

However, the work of some QNs gave cause for concern. Elizabeth Williams, who qualified as a QN in January 1907, left the Cheltenham DNA in July of the same year, after her first inspection found that it was "not desirable that Nurse Williams should be recommended again."[44] Hilda Boston was noted in 1924 to be "needing supervision" as her work was "rather slipshod." Eventually, she resigned from QVJI, when she was "cited to appear before CMB," her final inspection having found her to be "apt to neglect details. Very impulsive and has a difficult manner."[45] The Webb sisters were recognized as being kind and hardworking, and were liked by their patients, but Florence was considered "unsuitable for Public Health Work" and Lilian was "an unsatisfactory worker who needs strict supervision. Entirely unsuited for district midwifery and Child Welfare work." They served together as district nurses for only two years, at Cinderford in Gloucestershire from 1924 to 1926, before both resigned to take up private nursing.[46]

Improvements were acknowledged as a nurse's career progressed and she became more experienced and competent. Margaret Powell was "not up to Queen's standard" in 1906, but by the time she resigned from QVJI during World War I to take up a post as lady superintendent in a munitions factory, she was reported to be "an excellent School Nurse and a willing worker."[47] Kate Hastings was reported to be "not competent to teach" at Plaistow in 1908, but when she resigned her post in Manchester to be married in 1912, her final inspection found her to be "a very capable nurse with a good educational influence."[48]

Individual clashes of personality, regional traits, and a lack of knowledge of local customs could also cause problems. In such cases, comments could be blunt and unequivocal. Adeline Sproat left her first post in Northampton in 1908 because she "failed to work amicably with Supt," and in her next post in St. Helens, she was noted to have "not a happy disposition."[49] Caroline Lee was "hot-tempered, ... self-opinionated and impatient of control," while Susannah Jenkins was "not easy to get on with in the Home. . . . Quick-tempered, ... very difficult and over-bearing in manner."[50] Mildred Griffiths was noted to be "inexperienced in country work" in 1911, with a "somewhat irritating and self-opinionated manner."[51] Jessie Douglas was also "inexperienced in dealing with country people" when she took up her first post as a QN at Treverbyn in 1911, and while she was working at Gotherington in Gloucestershire from 1914 to 1915, her reports read "manner brusque, temperament lethargic" and "not very enthusiastic or sympathetic." However, when she returned to her native Scotland, she was reported to be "careful, interested and much-liked."[52] During twenty years as a QN in urban posts in the north of England, Catherine Phillips was regarded as "a clever, capable nurse," "a very careful maternity nurse and a pleasant woman," and "kind, willing to please." Yet, when she briefly worked at Nailsworth DNA in rural Gloucestershire in 1923, she was described by the honorary secretary as "untidy and unprincipled" and by the county superintendent as "unreliable and of a difficult temperament."[53] Rose Paling was "inclined to talk too much" and "resenting authority," while Beatrice Price was "somewhat secretive in manner."[54]

At the other extreme, an outstanding few progressed to senior positions within QVJI. Bessie Taylor was recognized during her district training to be "suitable for responsible post," and by 1920, she was county superintendent of the West Riding of Yorkshire, where she proved "equal to the work expected of her."[55] Lena Milford enjoyed an exemplary career in Gloucestershire as nurse at Coln St. Aldwyn, assistant county superintendent, and, from 1917 to 1946, "a wise, progressive, hard-working and highly esteemed" county superintendent.[56] With her forceful personality, Caroline Lee progressed to being county superintendent in Kent, Derbyshire, and Northamptonshire; she ended her career as a recruitment officer from 1930 to 1936, presenting "Queen's Institute Propaganda in Hospitals," where she was considered to be "an excellent speaker."[57]

The few district nurses who enjoyed such distinguished careers and rose to high office within QVJI could be said to be as unrepresentative and atypical a minority as were the negative examples. The silent majority of district nurses emerge from the Queen's Roll as unassuming and industrious workers who approached their duties with the loyalty and fortitude Florence Nightingale envisaged.

Lewis believes that midwifery and nursing both became middle-class preserves as the twentieth century progressed.[58] However, the evidence provided by the Queen's Roll suggests that district nursing, which combined midwifery and nursing, particularly in rural areas, increasingly attracted young women from the upper working classes. Furthermore, the statistic Lewis quotes, of 10 percent home deliveries in 1924, refers to all QVJI nurses; it does not differentiate between QNs and the second grade of district nurse that was introduced in rural areas.

Village Nurse-Midwives

The anomaly of rural district nursing lay in the fact that, in the areas where the nurses were most needed, the poor patients could least afford to subscribe to local funds, and many DNAs found themselves unable to pay the wage for a QN. In addition, many of the nurses were reluctant to work in isolated rural areas and found the responsibility of midwifery daunting. In an attempt to solve these problems, under the *Conditions of Affiliation for County Nursing Associations*, first issued in 1897 and revised in 1901, the Council of QVJI sanctioned "the employment of Village Nurses in rural districts where it is impossible to support a Queen's Nurse and the population of the district does not as a rule exceed 3,000."[59] These village nurse-midwives (VNMs), as they soon became known, were not hospital-trained nurses. They were local working-class women whose district and midwifery training was paid for by the CNA, in return for which they contracted to work in the county for a minimum of three years.

The introduction of this second grade of district nurse caused widespread resentment among the QNs, who regarded them as professionally inferior due to their lack of hospital experience. These feelings were made clear in an unattributed article in the *Queen's Nurses' Magazine* in 1910: "The work of County Nursing Associations is not very cordially accepted by many Queen's Nurses. There is a prevalent uneasy idea that the Queen's Institute in recognising these Associations and their 'Village Nurses' has departed from its original standard, and approves that much-scorned individual, the 'half-trained nurse'." The article reminded its readers that the supervision of VNMs by the county superintendent "had helped in a marked degree to raise the general standard of work" and reassured them that in rural areas, "where it is not possible to provide work and funds to justify the employment of a Queen's Nurse, the village nurse is a valuable factor, filling a real need, and under wise supervision taking her share in building up the health of the community."[60]

Despite the official support for VNMs, professional jealousy persisted among the district nurses. When Margaret Powell became an assistant superintendent to the Gloucestershire CNA, it was noted that she was "not always tactful in dealing with Village Nurses."[61] At a Conference of Queen's superintendents in 1913, "a lack of sisterly kindness on the part of some Queen's Nurses to their less trained sisters" was noted, and among the questions discussed was "Can we remove the spirit of opposition that exists in our midst against the employment of inferior trained nurses by County Associations?" Unfortunately, neither the points raised in the discussion nor the conclusion reached are recorded, but the fact that the matter was discussed at "one of the largest gatherings in the history of the association" illustrates both the extent of the problem and the seriousness with which it was regarded by the most senior members of QVJI.[62]

As a result of these concerns, over the years the length and content of training for VNMs were regularly reviewed and increased. In Gloucestershire, the first report of the CNA, dated 1905, specified that the qualifications for VNMs should be "Twelve months' – or in no case under six months' – training at some approved training place, with Midwifery instruction and certificate." The following year, it was stressed that the training of VNMs "forms one of the most important duties of the Association," but that this work had been "a good deal handicapped by lack of funds and the difficulty of finding suitable women to train as Village Nurses."[63] In fact, in April 1906, when the subcommittee responsible for selecting trainees "met at the Superintendent's house to interview candidates for training as Village Nurses, only one kept her appointment and she was not considered suitable."[64] Only two VNMs had completed their training that year and been appointed to DNAs in the county, Mathilda Brown, who "had started work at Sapperton & Coates and was much liked," and Jennie Chambers, who was reported to be "doing well at Whitminster." One candidate, Rose Gardiner, had broken down in health after three months training and had been sent home, and Miss Kendall, who had been interviewed and approved, regretted that "owing to private reasons" she could not accept the offer of training. A further two women, Mrs. Shaw and Letitia Burden, were in the course of training, while two candidates, Mrs. Roberts and Mrs. Till, had both twice failed to pass the CMB examination.

In 1906, QVJI increased the minimum training period for VNMs from six to nine months, and in 1909, a QVJI inspector informed the Gloucestershire CNA in her annual report of "the desirability of a twelve months' training for the County Nurses, as is now generally the rule," and as was laid down in the county's own scheme.[65] Implementation of these changes increased the cost of training for each nurse, an expense that had to be met from already stretched county funds, raised from grants, donations, subscriptions, and DNA affiliation fees, supplemented by parish collections, plant and garden sales, Flag days, and bazaars.

Between 1905 and 1919, the majority of Gloucestershire VNMs received their training at the District Nurses' Home at Plaistow in London, with the occasional placement of one or two trainees at the Victoria Home, Cheltenham, Kingswood in Bristol, or Tipton in the West Midlands. During that period, an average of six VNMs was trained each year. From 1919, Kingswood District Nurses' Home became the main training center for the county, although one or two trainees continued to be placed in Cheltenham. This arrangement "proved very satisfactory – the Home is very comfortable, and the pupils are thoroughly well trained and cared for in every way."

In 1907, the ideal VNM was described as a "young married woman who would be able to undertake the work in her own and neighbouring parishes."[66] However, the Gloucestershire CNA reports regularly express regret and concern at the great scarcity of suitable candidates for training. Unfortunately, few personal details are recorded of the VNM applicants, but from the available data it can be seen that the average age of candidates accepted for training was 31.3 years (see Table 2). When a year is added for training, the average age of qualifying as a VNM becomes 32.3 years. Of the seven applicants for whom marital status was recorded, one was single, one was separated, two were married, and three were widows. A further twenty-one applicants (not all of whom were accepted) are referred to in the CNA Minutes as "Mrs.," but whether they were married or widowed is not recorded.

Table 2.   Applicants Accepted for Training as VNMs in Gloucestershire

Year	Nurse's name	Background	Age
1905	Mrs. Till	Wife of a coachman	
1905	Jennie Chambers		38
1906	Letitia Burden	Separated, 1 child	26
1907	Alice O'Brian	Servant	
1908	Florence Bishop	Widow, no children	30
1908	Mrs. Dawe	Widow, 3 children	39
1908	Bessie Mourton	Single	35
1908	Mrs. Williams	Married, 2 children	35
1912	Chapman		26
1912	Florence Mann		27
1913	Taylor		24
1913	Vallender		33
1916	Mrs. Fitzgerald	Widow, 2 children (1 delicate)	

Source: GRO D2410.

Among the earliest applicants to be rejected was Mrs. Lucas, who "was 60 with no education and it was decided that it was impossible to help her," while Mrs. Edith Mills, aged forty-four, was considered "too old" and Mrs. Phillips "was quite of the cottage class."[67] Alice Brown was rejected in 1909, "as her medical certificate stated that her heart was not quite normal"; the following year, it was decided not to train Miss A. Hathaway, "as the doctor did not consider she was strong enough for district work"; and in 1911, Lizzie Hardwick was rejected "as her medical certificate was not satisfactory." Several women were classified as "unsatisfactory" or "not suitable" without any specific reason being given, including Mrs. Baxter, a widow from Cheltenham with six years experience as an unqualified midwife, and Mrs. Trigg, who had been approved in 1910, but "as further information had been received . . . it had been decided not to train [her]."

Among those who were approved for training, Minnie Bishop "wrote to say she did not wish to be trained as she could not bind herself to work in the County for three years," Bessie Mourton and Mathilda Wardle both fell ill and could not take up their training places, while Mrs. Loveday and Mrs. Laver both decided not to be trained. Nurse Thompson did complete her training in 1907, but her work at St. Briavels "was reported not to be very satisfactory." It was decided that the county superintendent "should talk to her and that she should be given another chance." She was transferred to a new district in January 1908, but after just two months in her new post, the secretary "wrote saying she had given Nurse Thompson notice as her work was not satisfactory. It was decided not to give her further employment." Fanny Wickenden was sent for training in August 1909, but she "did not appear equal to the demands made on her during the training and was recalled" in December.

In that same year, another Gloucestershire trainee, Mrs. Dawe, failed the CMB examination. The CNA Committee had clearly made a great effort to help Mrs. Dawe, a thirty-nine-year-old widow, as sufficient money had been subscribed to keep her three children for four months and "it was decided that if she was doing well in her training, steps would be taken for the other five months." However, the matron at the training home "did not give a good account of her capabilities ... [and] came to the conclusion she would have much to learn before she could pass an examination. The Committee decided not to continue Mrs. Dawe's training as they did not think she had the necessary qualities to make a good Village Nurse."

The VNMs were expected to pass the CMB examination, that is, the same midwifery qualification as QNs, who were already trained nurses. As we have seen, many QN candidates lacked the level of literacy this required, and the working-class VNM trainees encountered the same difficulties. This clearly caused a national problem, as in 1909, at a meeting of CNA representatives at QVJI's London offices, one of the subjects discussed was the need to simplify "the technical terms employed in the CMB examination."[68] In 1906, Margaret Loane, a distinguished QN, wrote a textbook, *Simple Introductory Lessons in Midwifery*, explaining medical terms. In the same year, the Gloucestershire CNA Committee agreed that Mrs. Shaw, in training at Plaistow, would have "6d per week sent to her for books, etc.," and in 1907, the county superintendent was authorized "to spend a sum of between 20/- and 30/- on books to be lent to pupils in training."[69]

Despite such help, candidates continued to struggle, and there are frequent references in the Gloucestershire CNA Minutes to nurses having to repeat the CMB examination. Nurse Conry managed to pass the written paper in June 1910, but failed the oral examination, which she passed at her second attempt a month later. Nurse Higgs and Nurse Harris both failed the CMB examination in August 1910 but passed in October. Nurse Aston passed at her second attempt in January 1913, while Nurse Sims only passed at her third attempt in February 1913. In 1912, "Nurse Burchill training at Plaistow was reported by the Superintendent to read and write so badly that it was feared she would not be able to pass the CMB examination. It was decided she should attend a night school while at Plaistow."

Other candidates failed to complete their training. Halfway through her course in 1910, Nurse Powis decided that "owing to family matters [she] did not wish to complete her training and re-paid the fees." In the same year, Nurse

Corkhill left Tipton after just one day "owing to her husband's illness. As she had stated that she was a single woman the Committee decided not to allow her to return." In 1911, Pearl Loveridge "returned home from Plaistow in bad health after 7 months training," while Mrs. Sinclair, having "left Plaistow during her training without permission, was interviewed by the Committee and promised to repay the sum spent on her."

Those who did complete their training were reported to have "all done well,"[70] and in 1910, the value of VNMs was stressed in the *Queen's Nurses Magazine*: "What they know, they know well – they are of the country, understand the people, and are happy amongst them.... Queen's Nurses are needed in increasing numbers, ... but under the pressure of the Midwives Act, ... the village nurses are also needed for the posts they alone can fill."[71]

The necessity of balancing the technical content of the training with the caliber of candidates remained a problem, particularly as the scope of their duties increased with the expansion of public health work after 1908. This involved health visiting, maternity and infant-welfare clinics, inspection of schoolchildren, and tuberculosis care. The nurses were expected to fulfill these duties in addition to their routine nursing and midwifery cases, and the VNMs were expected to carry the same weight of responsibility as QNs, despite their shorter training and lower wages.

The outbreak of World War I in 1914 also affected the recruitment of trainees, as many potential candidates took up war work in various capacities. In 1916, the Gloucestershire CNA noted that it was "very difficult to obtain candidates for training," and in 1917 a letter by the Duchess of Beaufort "calling attention to the need for women to train as District Nurses" was sent "to all the newspapers in the County."[72] By endorsing a similar national appeal by the president of the Hampshire CNA, the duchess acknowledged the "splendid desire ... [of] women to serve the country by war work," but she strongly recommended that, instead of "eagerly undertaking temporary employment where little training is necessary," women should consider training as VNMs and thus "fitting themselves to do permanent service for their country ... [as] an integral part of our health organisation."[73] The response to the original national appeal is not known, but in Gloucestershire twelve applications were received, although "some of these would not accept the conditions of training and some were not suitable but it is hoped 2 at least will be trained." Later that same year, "a letter was sent by the Secretary to all local associations asking if they could recommend candidates for training," but only two women applied.[74]

At that time, Gloucestershire VNMs were given "careful instruction" in health work by the county superintendent as part of her supervisory duties, but at a Conference of Superintendents in London in 1919, it was considered desirable that such instruction should become an integral part of their training.[75] At the Conference of Superintendents in 1922, a resolution was passed "to the effect that the period of training for Village Nurses should be extended to one and a half years, and that three months of that time should, if possible, be devoted to school work and health visiting."[76] In Gloucestershire, an extra three months instruction in health work was added to the one year's training in 1922/3, and in 1925/6, it was reported that the county's VNMs "will now receive eighteen months training, one year in Midwifery and six months in general and Health work" and "to bind for a period of two years instead of three."[77]

In 1924–5, the Gloucestershire CNA reported that, although the number of applicants had increased, "very few of these are suitable for the work."[78] A breakdown in health was still the most frequently cited reason for candidates failing to complete their training: Nurse Prince at Kingswood in 1920; Nurse Markham after only a fortnight's training in 1921; Nurse Wilkins, who had been at Kingswood for three months in 1923; Nurse Hepburn, who spent sixteen weeks in training at the Victoria Home, Cheltenham, also in 1923; and Nurse Smallbones, who broke her contract at the end of three months training in 1924, "being too nervous for the work."[79] In 1925, it was recorded that "it has not been possible to keep the vacancies at Kingswood filled during the whole year," and the CNA expressed "regret and surprise that many more women do not feel a vocation to a life so full of human interest and personal devotion."[80] However, in a paper delivered at the Conference of Superintendents in 1922, Miss Johnson, the county superintendent for the Isle of Wight, pointed out that with the implementation of the Registration Act, "the most eminently suitable women would consider the county training not worth while" because, on the completion of her training, each candidate "will *not* be a fully qualified nurse . . . [and] she will be unable to come into any scheme for the benefit of fully trained nurses."[81] In Gloucestershire, attempts were made to recognize the quality and professionalism of the VNMs by the introduction, in 1919, of a certificate "for nurses leaving the County after fulfilling their contract and having worked satisfactorily," and in 1920, by the wearing of a county badge: a white enameled badge during a nurse's first two years of service, then "if satisfactory," a red badge.[82]

Despite such ongoing problems and concerns, VNMs remained invaluable. In England and Wales as a whole, they represented 25.44 percent of QVJI nurses in 1905; by 1925, this figure had risen to 62.38 percent, a percentage increase of 36.94. In Gloucestershire, a predominantly rural county, VNMs as a percentage of QVJI nurses rose from 57.14 in 1907 to 82.44 in 1925. In a report dated 1926, the county medical officer of health described how "much useful work has been done by the District Nurses in the County and the value of their services as health agencies in the homes becomes more obvious as time goes on. It is scarcely stating too much to say that there is no other service which has such full opportunity for promoting the general health of the country, for the home is the unit of health work, and the District Nurse enters it more intimately than can any other health official."[83]

> Although professional resentment persisted nationally, in Gloucestershire the dual system of QNs and VNMs, both combining district nursing with health work, was clearly a success, and in its report of 1925/6, the Gloucestershire CNA recorded with pride that "the combination of State and Voluntary Work as carried out in this County is held up as a model all over the Country."[84]

Conclusion

The work of rural district nurses demanded skill, tact, and stamina, if they were to achieve their dual aims of improving the lives of their working-class patients and caring for them. Although the QNs were expected to be "ladies," the Queen's Roll suggests that, initially, district work appealed more to young women from a middle-class background and by the interwar period was attracting candidates from the upper working classes. Although, as a consequence, educational difficulties were frequently cited as a cause for concern, QVJI's demanding training, unique system of inspections, and centrally held records provided the means to carefully monitor each nurse from her initial training to each post she subsequently held. Hence, any problems were identified, recorded, and dealt with to ensure standards were maintained.

Poor literary skills were also a major problem in the recruitment and training of VNMs, with many candidates having to repeat the CMB examination before they passed at the second or even third attempt. Poor health prevented some candidates from even completing their training and those who did qualify found themselves excluded by the Registration Act of 1919. However, the VNMs represented an integral and invaluable part of the national rural district nursing scheme, and the organizational structure of QVJI remained unchanged until it was absorbed into the NHS in 1948.

Those nurses, both QNs and VNMs, who did prove suitable for rural district work derived a great sense of satisfaction and social status from their combined duties of nursing, midwifery, and public health work. In late nineteenth- and early-twentieth-century hospitals, all patients were referred to by their bed number, and nurses were frequently changed from side to side in a ward to prevent them from getting to know any patient too well. It was also traditional to call senior nurses by the names of their wards (e.g., Sister Clinical) instead of by their own surnames.[85] In contrast to such an impersonal atmosphere, rural district nursing offered the opportunity to befriend entire families and to occupy a position of trust and respect within the community.

Among the QNs who served in Gloucestershire, where the rural movement began, Alpha Fenton worked at Charlton Kings for seventeen years and her successor, Ann Newdick, for twenty-four years; Rose Paling worked at Lydney for sixteen years, Beatrice Price at Stone for eighteen years, and Lucy Avery at Nailsworth for twenty-four years. Among the longest-serving VNMs in the county, Nurses Shaw, Kite, Self, and Fitzgerald were already either married or widowed when they began their training, while two of the longest-serving QNs remained in their posts after marriage, Nurse Price becoming Mrs. Pullir in 1927 and Nurse Avery becoming Mrs. Abbotts in 1936. VNM Nurse Bridges, who worked for the Coln St. Aldwyn DNA from 1917 to 1927, was allowed to continue in her post when she became Mrs. Day in 1922, when she informed the committee that "she would like to settle down" in the area.[86] Similarly, VNMs Nurse Hill, appointed to Kings Stanley in 1919, and Nurse Cooper, appointed to Wotton-under-Edge in the same year, both remained in the same posts when they married in 1925, becoming Mrs. Miles and Mrs. Witchell, respectively. This, of course, was in marked contrast to hospital nurses, who were expected to resign on marriage, and it must have been an inducement to those who wanted to combine a family life with paid service to the community of which they had become an integral part.

In evaluating the success of the district nurses, it must be remembered that QVJI was a charity and the poor were not obliged to use its services. The Midwives Act of 1902 forbade the practice of midwifery other than by trained and registered women, but no such act was passed to prevent unqualified attendance to the sick and dying. The fact that the rural district nurses overcame deeply entrenched local customs and prejudices and established themselves as part of village life is a testament to the self-effacing and hardworking majority and, clearly, the nursing, midwifery, and health care they provided was welcome. However, the success of the educational aspects of QVJI's aims is more difficult to quantify or qualify. During the late nineteenth and early twentieth centuries, policy makers, social investigators, and philanthropists paid increasing attention to the problems of poor families and subjected them to increasingly close supervision. Concern over the poor physical condition of army recruits during the Boer War between Britain and the Dutch colonists in South Africa (1899–1902) had generated a national campaign to improve the health and welfare of the young, but government intervention was limited by the accepted belief that family responsibilities provided the best and greatest incentives for men to work. Even after the Insurance Act of 1911 and the provision of the first sickness and maternity benefits, successive governments resisted calls for further direct economic assistance, such as family allowances. As one of the main agencies of care and health education, the scope of QVJI's services was, therefore, confined within government policies that were designed to inculcate a sense of moral responsibility without increasing the financial burden of the country's economy by directly relieving the problems of poverty and poor living conditions.

Nevertheless, the poor recognized and appreciated the advantages of the professional care that QVJI's nurses could offer. At Upton St. Leonards in Gloucestershire in 1908, the county superintendent reported that Nurse Goddard "is loved by her patients . . . [and] it was a pleasure to go round the district with her,"[87] while at Gotherington in 1911, Elizabeth Malleson noted that "Nurse Griffiths has already won her place amongst us by her habitual manner of regarding patients not only as 'cases' in nursing parlance, but as neighbours and friends requiring her skilled help."[88] Mary Paget, who was delivered by Nurse Ann Newdick at Charlton Kings on a Sunday morning in 1912, recalls, "She was absolutely wonderful and much respected in the village."[89] Alexina Cowee was "a kind, unselfish and attentive nurse. Much liked."[90] Lily Tatton was "conscientious and hard-working, kind and with a gentle manner,"[91] and Lucy Avery was "a keen and energetic nurse, much appreciated by doctors and patients."[92] At Nailsworth in 1920, it was recorded that "the Nurse is welcomed everywhere."[93] By 1924, the Gloucestershire CNA was "particularly glad to be able to report that . . . the desire to have a Nurse in practically every parish comes from the people themselves, and is a gratifying proof that the quiet devoted work of the Nurses in the homes for the past twenty years and more is bearing fruit."[94]

The appreciation felt by the poor was often displayed by simple but touching gestures. One of QVJI's most stringent rules was that "the nurse shall not accept any presents from patients or their friends,"[95] but at Upton St. Leonards in 1907, the DNA Committee found it necessary to modify this rule by the addition of the clause "other than flowers or fruit."[96] At Gotherington in 1913, Elizabeth Malleson recorded that "one suffering woman on her death-bed begged that the Nurse might be asked to accept the gift of one of her possessions as a token of her care and help; such a gift was against official rules, but in my mind such a wish left no obligation but obedience to it."[97] The DNA Committee at Nailsworth was also willing to interpret the rule flexibly, as it was noted in 1925 that Nurse Avery "frequently tells the Committee members that on her return home from work she finds on her doorstep gifts of a few plants, flowers, a few eggs, a pot of jam, and similar marks of gratitude from an appreciative public."[98]

Overall, QVJI failed to attract the class of recruits that its founders and leaders originally envisaged, particularly in rural areas, where it proved necessary to introduce a second grade of nurse. The district nurses did take a greater level and scope of care into the homes of the rural poor than had ever been available to them before, but although the services they offered did much to relieve the effects of poverty, social policies failed to solve the underlying causes. Nevertheless, with its combination of home nursing, midwifery, and public health work, and its national system of inspections and centrally held ongoing records, rural district nursing, more than any other branch of the profession, came closest to fulfilling Florence Nightingale's vision of the future of nursing, while the nurses themselves, both QNs and VNMs, whether single, married, or widowed, could live as part of a community in which their work was rewarded with the hard-won respect, affection, and gratitude of their poor patients.

CARRIE HOWSE, BED (HON), MA, PHD
External Member
University of Gloucestershire
30 Rothleigh
Up Hatherley
Cheltenham
Glos GL51 3PS
England

Notes

1. For example, see the two classic texts on nursing in England, Brian Abel-Smith, *A History of the Nursing Profession* (London: Heinemann, 1960) and Christopher Maggs, *The Origins of General Nursing* (Beckenham, Kent: Croom Helm, 1983).

2. Mary Stocks, *A Hundred Years of District Nursing* (London: Allen & Unwin, 1960); Monica Baly, *A History of the Queen's Nursing Institute* (Beckenham, Kent: Croom Helm, 1987). The title QVJI was changed in 1928 to the Queen's Institute of District Nursing and later still to the Queen's Nursing Institute. Throughout this article, which covers the years 1880 to 1925, the original title is used.

3. Baly, *History of the Queen's Nursing Institute,* flyleaf.

4. Cecil Woodham-Smith, *Florence Nightingale* (1950; reprint London: Book Club Associates, 1972), 539.

5. Stocks, *District Nursing,* 43.

6. Florence Nightingale, Letter, *The Times,* April 14, 1876, page 6.

7. *The Lancet,* April 22, 1876, pp. 610–11.

8. Nightingale, Letter, April 14, 1876.

9. *The Lancet,* April 22, 1876, pp. 610–11.

10. Nightingale, Letter, April 14, 1876.

11. *The Lancet,* April 22, 1876, pp. 610–11.

12. F.K. Prochaska, *Women and Philanthropy in Nineteenth Century England* (Oxford: Oxford University Press, 1980), 98.

13. Rosalind Nash, ed., *Florence Nightingale to Her Nurses: A Selection from Miss Nightingale's Addresses to Probationers and Nurses of the Nightingale School at St. Thomas' Hospital, 1872–1888* (London: Macmillan, 1914), 45–7.

14. Baly, *Queen's Nursing Institute,* 31–2.

15. Gwen Hardy, *William Rathbone and the Early History of District Nursing* (Ormskirk, Lancs: Hesketh, 1981), 49.

16. See Carrie Howse, "The Development of Rural District Nursing in Gloucestershire, 1880–1925," PhD thesis, University of Gloucestershire, 2004.

17. Committee of QVJI, Letter, *The Times,* January 7, 1888, page 8.

18. Editorial, *The Times,* January 7, 1888, page 9.

19. F.R.C.S., Letter, *The Times,* January 18, 1888, page 9; Isaac Butler, Letter, *The Times,* January 21, 1888, page 4.

20. Florence Nightingale, "Sick-Nursing and Health-Nursing," in Baroness Angela Burdett-Coutts, ed., *Woman's Mission: A Series of Congress Papers on the Philanthropic Work of Women by Eminent Writers* (London: Sampson Low, Marston, 1893), p. 186.

21. Nightingale, "Sick Nursing," p. 192–4.

22. Nightingale, "Sick Nursing," p. 195.

23. Nightingale, "Sick Nursing," p. 200.

24. Florence Craven, *A Guide to District Nurses and Home Nursing* (1889; reprint London: Macmillan, 1894), 1–6.

25. Gloucestershire Record Office, D4057/14 (hereafter GRO).

26. Jane Lewis, *The Politics of Motherhood: Child and Maternal Welfare in England, 1900–1939* (London: Croom Helm, 1980), 121, 144, 142.

27. GRO D2410.

28. See Carrie Howse, "Registration: A Minor Victory?" *Nursing Times,* 85, no. 49 (December 1989): 32–4.

29. Woodham-Smith, *Nightingale,* 571–3.

30. Contemporary Medical Archives Centre, Wellcome Institute, London, The Queen's Roll, SA/QNI/J.3/2 (hereafter CMAC).

31. CMAC SA/QNI/J.3/9-15.

32. Unattributed, "The Conference of Queen's Superintendents," *Queen's Nurses' Magazine,* 10, Part 2 (April 1913): 35–47 (hereafter *QNM*).

33. CMAC SA/QNI/J.3/17-23.

34. Unattributed, "Report of Queen's Superintendents' Annual Conference," *QNM,* 19, Part 2 (1922): 25–29.

35. CMAC SA/QNI/J.3/24-31.

36. CMAC SA/QNI/J.3/23.

37. Martha Vicinus, *Independent Women: Work and Community for Single Women, 1850–1920* (London: Virago, 1985), 109–16.

38. GRO D2774 3/1.

39. GRO D2465 4/32–33.
40. CMAC SA/QNI/J.3/11.
41. *QNM,* 19, Part 2 (1922): 30.
42. *QNM,* 19, Part 2 (1922): 28.
43. CMAC SA/QNI/J.3/2, 9, 10.
44. CMAC SA/QNI/J.3/13.
45. CMAC SA/QNI/J.3/24.
46. CMAC SA/QNI/J.3/30.
47. CMAC SA/QNI/J.3/13.
48. CMAC SA/QNI/J.3/10.
49. CMAC SA/QNI/J.3/15.
50. CMAC SA/QNI/J.3/17; CMAC SA/QNI/J.3/29.
51. CMAC SA/QNI/J.3/18.
52. CMAC SA/QNI/J.3/18.
53. CMAC SA/QNI/J.3/10.
54. CMAC SA/QNI/J.3/19; CMAC SA/QNI/J.3/23.
55. CMAC SA/QNI/J.3/15.
56. CMAC SA/QNI/J.3/17.
57. CMAC SA/QNI/J.3/17.
58. Lewis, *Motherhood,* 145.
59. GRO D4057/14.
60. Unattributed, "County Nursing Associations and Their Work," *QNM,* 7, Part 1 (1910): 9–11.
61. CMAC SA/QNI/J.3/13.
62. *QNM,* 10, Part 2 (1913): 36.
63. GRO D4057/1.
64. GRO D2410.
65. GRO D4057/1.
66. GRO D4057/1.
67. GRO D2410.
68. GRO D4057/1.
69. GRO D2410.
70. GRO D4057/1.
71. *QNM,* 7, Part 1 (1910): 10.
72. GRO D2410.
73. *Gloucestershire Echo,* April 9, 1917.
74. GRO D2410.
75. GRO D2410.
76. *QNM,* 19 Part 2 (1922): 27.
77. GRO D4057/1; GRO D2410.
78. GRO D4057/1.
79. GRO D2410.
80. GRO D4057/1.
81. *QNM,* 19, Part 2 (1922): 29–30.
82. GRO D2410.
83. GRO D4057/6.
84. GRO D4057/1.

85. Vicinus, *Independent Women,* 107; Judith Moore, *A Zeal for Responsibility: The Struggle for Professional Nursing in Victorian England, 1868–1883* (Athens: University of Georgia Press, 1988), 58.

86. Hicks-Beach private family papers, courtesy of Lord St. Aldwyn.

87. GRO P347 MI 3/1.

88. GRO D4057/15.

89. Interview, January 17, 2003.

90. CMAC SA/QNI/J.3/11.

91. CMAC SA/QNI/J.3/18.

92. CMAC SA/QNI/J.3/31.

93. GRO D3548 3/1.

94. GRO D4057/1.

95. GRO D4057/3.

96. GRO P347 MI 3/1.

97. GRO D4057/15.

98. GRO D3548 3/1.

"Much Instruction Needed Here": The Work of Nurses in Rural Wisconsin During the Depression

RIMA D. APPLE
University of Wisconsin–Madison

In October 1936, Mildred Cook was looking for an address in Pulaski, Wisconsin. In the process, Cook, a nurse working for the State of Wisconsin Bureau of Maternal and Child Health, came across Mrs. J.B. This woman was pregnant and due in March, but she had not yet seen her doctor. Cook urged her to do so. The next day the nurse was gratified to learn that the woman had followed her advice and visited the physician. Moreover, she was proud to announce that "Doctor was very pleased with this work."[1] Through her counsel, Cook had accomplished two important goals of the State Department of Health. She had convinced a client of the importance of prenatal medical examinations, and she had cemented a particularly positive relationship with the local physician. Cook's work illustrates the epitome of maternal health care throughout most of the twentieth century in the United States: physician supervised, nurse assisted, medically directed.

Cook was a critical actor in a unique public health experiment, a joint effort that linked federal, state, and county governments and community members in an innovative program to improve maternal and child health in rural Wisconsin. Concern for the welfare of mothers, pregnant women, and young children led many governmental agencies and philanthropic organizations to develop programs to alleviate health and nutrition problems that were exacerbated by the worsening economic conditions of the Depression. In Wisconsin, the Department of Health instituted the Demonstration Nurse Program in which the state Bureau of Maternal and Child Health used federal dollars to hire public health nurses to work in rural counties. Most critically, this program was time limited. The state health officials planned to fund these nurses only for a year or two, after which they expected that the counties would recognize the advantages of county nurses and begin to employ these women with local funding. In other words, the goal was that the County Demonstration Nurses would *demonstrate* the efficacy of public health nurses.

This situation placed nurses like Cook in a precarious position. As state employees, the nurses needed to follow the state program. As public health nurses, they needed to assure local physicians that the state was not interfering with private medical practice. As demonstration nurses, they needed to develop positive health statistics for the county. As frontline health care workers, they needed to improve the health and well-being of their clients and their children. This balancing of the various, at times competing, aspects of the position was difficult to maintain and could be torturous for the nurse. When she originally arrived in Barron County in February 1940, Louise Steffen, RN, assiduously cultivated physicians, county board members, township offices, and other community leaders, who generally agreed that a county nurse was needed and even offered their support. Yet, it was not until November 1943 that the County Board appropriated the funds; in December, Hazel Nordley, who had succeeded Steffen as demonstration nurse, was named County Nurse in Barron County.[2] In Barron and some other counties, the nurses succeeded in convincing officials to fund the position; in other counties, officials declined to pick up the nurse's salary.

This article is part of a larger study that will analyze the factors that contributed to the success of the program in some counties and that led to its demise in others. Here, I focus on the daily work of the County Demonstration Nurses in order to understand the tensions inherent in their positions and the factors that inhibited and encouraged their practices.[3] I examine the day-to-day activities of frontline public health workers who consistently admonished women to use modern scientific medical discoveries in caring for their families. The nurses prepared statistical studies to provide quantitative evidence of their work and their successes, numbers for the Bureau to use to argue for the employment of a permanent county nurse. In addition, they wrote detailed narrative reports, describing their daily experiences and interactions with patients, physicians, and local officials, as well as expressing their frustrations with local conditions and their pride in their accomplishments. With these data, they expected the Bureau to help them through the labyrinth of local politics. Through the pens and typewriters of nurses such as Cook and Steffens, we can begin to see the strategies of public health nurses who sought to bring modern science and medicine to mothers, while coping with the strictures of the U.S. medical system—specifically, the separation of "public health" and "private medicine."

Concern for High Rates of Infant and Maternal Mortality

Infant and maternal health statistics are critical indicators of the well-being of a nation. In the early years of the twentieth century, particularly in the industrialized countries of the West, high rates of infant and maternal mortality were lamented as adversely affecting national prestige and threatening economic and political power. This was not strictly a question of population growth; that is, the U.S. population in this era grew due, in part, to successive waves of immigration, primarily from Europe. It was, rather, the question of a healthy population.[4] Although scattered local efforts to reverse rising numbers of infant and maternal deaths were initiated in the United States in the nineteenth century, it was in the interwar period that health care providers, social reformers, educators, and politicians joined in a concerted effort to improve maternal and child health.

Identifying the critical role of mothers in this endeavor, their campaigns were designed to educate women in "modern," appropriate child care practices, such as precise scheduling, dietary supplements such as cod liver oil, and regular medical check-ups. This advice was predicated on middle-class standards for urban families that had the financial and medical resources to carry out such health care prescriptions.[5] Urban mothers who could not afford to attend a private physician were urged to visit the clinics that were being developed in cities such as New York, Chicago, and Milwaukee. The "ideal mother" embraced the increasing intervention of medical and scientific expertise and experts in her childrearing.[6]

The shame of the high rates of infant and maternal mortality galvanized social reformers at the turn of the twentieth century.[7] In reaction to the nation's concern, the U.S. Children's Bureau was established in 1912, with a mandate to "investigate and report . . . upon all matters pertaining to the welfare of children and child life among all classes of our people." Note that the agency was to investigate and report, not treat; yet, within its limited charge, the Bureau accomplished much in its first years, under the direction of Julia Lathrop, a former resident of Hull House in Chicago. It conducted well-publicized studies that highlighted the connections between infant and maternal mortality and morbidity and poverty in rural and urban areas. It produced popular childrearing brochures for general distribution to mothers across the country, among them *Prenatal Care* (1913) and *Infant Care* (1914), which proved to be the most popular of all the federal publications.

Yet, reformers bridled at the limitations of an agency that could do no more than conduct studies and publish brochures.[8] They also pushed for enactment of the Sheppard-Towner Act, which passed in 1921 despite powerful medical opposition.[9] To placate physicians who feared that Sheppard-Towner would lead to state medicine, the drafters carefully distinguished between health education, which was publicly financed, and medical care, which was between patient and physician. The act sanctioned and strengthened the boundaries between public health and private practice by providing matching grants to states restricted to information and instruction in nutrition and hygiene and prenatal and child health clinics. These activities clearly differentiated public health, such as clinics that would *detect* disease conditions, and private medical practice, construed as the *treatment* of disease conditions.[10]

Wisconsin's Reactions

Wisconsin initially used the federal funds to build the Wisconsin Child Health Special, a trailer staffed by Bureau nurses and physicians that moved from village to town to crossroads, offering health clinics in rural areas. As Sheppard-Towner funds declined toward the end of the 1920s, the work of the Wisconsin Child Health Special was augmented by health clinics sponsored by local philanthropic and service organizations, again staffed by Bureau nurses and physicians. With the passage of the Social Security Act of 1935, the state's nurses expanded their educational program and well-child clinics and added an important new dimension to their work: home visits to pregnant women, new mothers, and children.

Because of the sharp demarcation between public health and private medicine, state public health physicians conducted their work in temporary health centers. They saw the clients who attended the centers, and although some clients attempted to attend every center available, the centers themselves were held infrequently in any given location. How often centers could be held was affected in large part by the support of local service and philanthropic organizations, such as the Auxiliary of the American Legion, Women's Christian Temperance Union, Red Cross, and Homemakers Club. Other influential factors included resistance of local physicians, public health nurses' and physicians' perceptions of local needs, and local environmental conditions. For example, it quickly became apparent that attendance would be significantly lower during the harvest season. Because of the clinics' irregular schedule, physicians rarely developed continuing relationships with the clients or the community, and their reports back to the Bureau were often brief.

Identifying Clients

The nurses held a different position, and their reports were significantly fuller as they actively searched the community to identify potential clients even before assistance was requested. Nearly all the nurses related stories about finding patients while simply driving about the area. Grace M. Connors wrote with particular delight in October 1936: "Mrs H: Saw baby washing on the line. Peeked at mail box for name, and went in, and lo and behold she was expecting me, as she had heard that I called on all new babies. Was I glad ever that I had taken the name from the mail box, so that I could call her by name. She had two preschoolers also, and had a number of questions saved up to ask. I find quite a few families by watching for washings on lines on my way to and from some place."[11] The nurses often served as intermediaries between local physicians and clients. They visited clients in their homes, where they noted domestic conditions that could limit successful application of medical advice. They lived in the community. Yet, they were always aware that they stood in an educational, advisory role, subordinate to that of the physician.

Some of the nurses were comfortable in this environment, and their reports radiate a commitment and a passion for their work and their patients. While not glossing over rural problems, especially during the Depression Era, Connors wrote with an enthusiasm and even humor about the people she met. On August 1, 1936, she "Stopped by to see Dr. Andrew at Plainfield, just for old time's sake. . . . He referred a Mrs. W to me. He had just called there the day before, because the baby just didn't 'act right.' He found they were giving three day old baby sour milk. Visited Mrs. W. 'Well, the cows are in the marsh 2 miles away. By the time they milk them and walk two miles in this hot weather, it is turned a bit.' I found baby getting orange juice but it seemed to agree better than the sour milk!"[12]

Although committed to providing modern medical advice, Connors realized that many mothers had to be led slowly to new methods and ideas and worked with the local physicians to provide them. In one particularly poignant October 1936 case, she reflected: "Mrs. L reported by neighbor – twin boys, 1 mo old, makes 4 children and the oldest will not be 3 until Christmas Day. . . . Much instruction needed here, but I'll have to go easy, give a little at a time."[13] In contrast, the reports of another nurse, who worked in northwestern Wisconsin, are brusque. Compliant patients were discussed only briefly: "Sept 2 [1937:] Mrs. T – has everything ready for home delivery. Model patient; has done exactly as she was told." Patients who did not fit this picture were described very differently. In June 1937, she visited Mrs. S.H., a Native American. D., Mrs. H's daughter, had "delivered of her second illegitimate child seven weeks ago," at which time D. had been diagnosed with tuberculosis and sent to a hospital for Native Americans in northern Wisconsin. On June 21, the nurse "found our dear [D] at home saying she ran away from the hospital because the nurses insulted her. I tried to tell her she must return and to instruct her as best I could how to care for herself until she could be taken back. This is a difficult family to deal with because both [D] and her mother are such dreadful liars."[14]

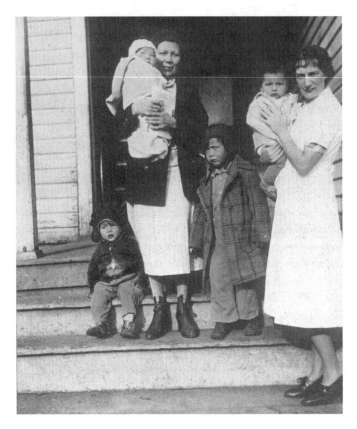

Figure 1. A nurse posed with a Native American mother and her four children in the 1930s. Reprinted courtesy of the Wisconsin Historical Society.

Often at the beginning of their work, the nurses grumbled about the problems identifying potential patients and the resistance they met from defensive and wary residents. Most soon found clients anxious for their advice, however, and resistance waned. Connors confessed in October 1936, "I want them to want me, and not to have to sort of throw myself at them. But I believe in due time it will work out O.K."[15] Her later reports clearly document her success in reaching the mothers of central Wisconsin.

As she was leaving her position in Marinette County in 1942, Nathalie Voge probably summed up the sentiments of many of the state's nurses: "The baby in a box of rags; a rusty barrel for a stove; no windows; rain leaking through the roof; two rooms and eight children; and the chickens picking at the bread which is rising on the table.... There are many a day when I would return home wondering, 'Will I ever be able to teach that family anything?' And then there were days when I thought a Public Health Nurse had the best job in the world. . . ."

Each day a county nurse brings joy, sorrow, and always something new and unexpected, but all in all the joy greatly outweighs the sorrows.[16] At any rate, because of the different personalities of the report writers and the variety of conditions they faced in rural Wisconsin, their narrative reports should be read not as representative but rather as emblematic of their time and place. Whether optimistic or pessimistic, the nurses of the Bureau of Maternal and Child Health conscientiously brought the message of good health to the mothers of rural Wisconsin while treading a fine line between treatment and preventive medicine.

A nurse began her work identifying pregnant women, new mothers, and preschool children in her territory. If another nurse had preceded her, she could start with the records of previous patients. Nurses also made follow-up visits to mothers who had attended one of the state-run health centers. Alternatively, as Connors's example of Mrs. W. demonstrates, local physicians could and did make referrals. When they did, nurses were careful to reinforce the messages women received from physicians. Nurses were careful to maintain a positive relationship with local doctors. On entering a community, the nurse would attempt to visit all the local physicians individually to discuss the program and the Standing Orders under which the nurses usually worked.[17] Physicians could either endorse the Standing Orders or modify them as necessary for their practices. Despite these efforts, some physicians continued to fear the loss of patients. Nurses sought to reassure medical practitioners that they were there to support, not detract from, the practice of the private physician.

Medical referrals were only a limited source of potential patients for these nurses. Nurses also combed through newly registered birth and death certificates to locate infants and mothers. As in the case of Mrs. L., they often learned of impending and recent births from neighbors. Hazel Nordley, who worked in northern Wisconsin in 1940, found that neighbors were crucial. Moreover, Nordley recognized that the early days following birth are critical "teaching moments": "The mothers have so many questions to ask about the new babies and it always seems as if there is so much information to be given at this time." Therefore, she devised a unique system for reaching new mothers promptly in the area; she distributed to each pregnant woman she saw a mimeographed postcard, asking her to complete and mail the card immediately after birthing. Mothers appreciated her consideration and, within months of beginning the program, Nordley reported that many of the cards were being returned quickly.[18] Nurses were also called on to lecture for a local Homemakers Council, Girl Scout troop, or high school class. They used these opportunities to identify other potential patients in the community. In addition to these specific actions designed to locate pregnant women, new mothers, and young children, there was also serendipity, such as Cook's finding Mrs. J.B. in Pulaski.

Conditions of Rural Life

Nurses would sometimes write about better-off, better-educated women. In Taylor, a town in western Wisconsin, in 1938, the nurse was pleased to report about her visit with Mrs. H.O. Mr. O. was principal of the school in Taylor, and the family had a two-and-a-half-month-old daughter. Significantly, Mrs. O. had been reading and carefully following the instruction in *Infant Care*; her baby was breastfed on a regular schedule and given cod liver oil and orange juice daily. Both regularity of feeding and the administration of cod liver oil and orange juice were keynotes of the advice of state nurses, reflective of the advice in much of the popular and medical literature of the day. Not surprisingly, the nurse had a high opinion of this case: "Baby is apparently on an ideal schedule and appears to be in excellent condition."[19]

But more often, reports from nurses were filled with sad stories of lack of resources, lack of knowledge, and lack of emotion and energy. Typical was a 1940 case in Marathon County in north-central Wisconsin. Through county relief, the family received two quarts of milk a day for eight children. The mother allocated one and a half quarts to the two youngest children, but the family had no eggs, fruit, or vegetables.[20] In another case, a visit to a Black River Falls family in western Wisconsin disclosed that the mother was out picking blueberries, leaving a five-month-old baby in the care of a blind grandmother. The baby slept in a large bed with a bottle propped beside her. There were flies everywhere. "Explained to grandmother that flies were disease carriers, and every effort should be made to keep the flies away from the baby," the nurse wrote later. "Grandmother said this was very difficult as there are no screen doors and the screens on the windows are very poor." In this case, the mother had won $5 in a community drawing and was planning to purchase a baby carriage with some of the winnings. The nurse advised them to buy the carriage and also netting to cover the baby to protect her from flies.[21] Nurses would find homes of Native Americans, Polish and Irish immigrants, and native-born residents where women were to deliver shortly where the ramshackle houses lacked basic utilities and the women lacked the most rudimentary elements of layette and supplies for home birth. Connors cogently explained why many women were not getting prenatal care: "Cannot pay M.D. any more than $15.00 and that is on time. Relief pays only $15.00 for delivery. M.D. can'st [sic] have anywhere from 8 to 16 prenatal visits, delivery, driving anywhere from 5 to 40 miles, post-natal visits, and postnatal examinations for $15.00 a case and not lost [sic] money. These mothers can't have proper food, cod liver oil, and calcium."[22] Lack of economic resources in many cases made it difficult for these rural women and their children to heed the well-meaning advice of the public health nurses who visited them, much less follow the recommendation to visit a physician.

Frequently, nurses described the trials and tribulations of simply reaching potential patients. Steffen wrote with concern that many families lived on country roads that made them difficult to reach. She astutely remarked, "The conditions of the roads [are] nothing new to the residents of the country, but [are] very new to me."[23] Catherine McLetchie colorfully recounted making a call on a family living deep in the woods: "It was necessary to leave the car at a neighbors, and walk through several fields, in one of which a bull was tethered. He seemed only mildly interested in the nurse, who luckily was wearing blue, not red! After walking through woods, up and down hills, and crawling under two fences, in twenty minutes or so the house was reached. Then the whole process was repeated on the return journey. It was a very hot, tired, and perspiring nurse that finally reached the car and relaxed somewhat behind the wheel."[24]

Although written from the perspective of nurses who understood that traveling conditions impeded their ability to delivery optimal health care, such reports are indicative of the problems faced by rural families as well. If public health nurses had difficulty getting to these women and their children, how likely was it that a private physician would make frequent calls? That food and other supplies could be delivered regularly and easily? That families could maintain easy contact with the larger world?

Bringing the Message of Good Health

But despite these geographic and economic obstacles, or perhaps because of them, many mothers were eager to hear about the latest medical advice and be reassured by medical professionals that their children were healthy and normal. Particularly popular were bath demonstrations. Nordley found that among young mothers, "this service is appreciated a great deal" and even "mothers who have children have asked for the bath demonstration."[25] Ruth Exner, in Grant County in 1940, made special efforts to speak to mothers in the early postpartum period because she realized that "young mothers are anxious to learn simpler ways of taking care of their new babies. One thing in particular is the baby's bath tray which has appealed to so many."[26] Given the resource demands of this "appropriate" infant bath, involving sterile cotton, separate washcloth and basin, special "mild baby soap," and the like, and its time demands, it is doubtful that many of the poor, exhausted mothers could continue similar routines daily.[27] Yet, whether they could follow through on the nurse's instructions or merely wanted to have another pair of hands helping in the family, mothers' interest in infant bathing indicates the value they placed on the assistance of health care experts.

Moreover, many nurses apparently used the demonstration of a bath as an opening wedge to initiate discussion of other aspects of child care. Thelma Burke understood that a mother could use this practical instruction to learn more. "I've given one infant demonstration bath where the mother 'fired' questions at me," she reported from north-central Wisconsin. "If I can get over the road, I'll return next week to see how much they have been able to follow." Although this young mother was eager to hear about modern concepts, Burke despaired of her practicing them because "Since Grandma, who came from Poland, lives there too, it might be very difficult for the mother to do what she really wants."[28]

Despite their attempted rapport with their patients, there were times nurses simply could not comprehend the lives of these struggling rural women or why they did not embrace modern medical care. At the beginning of November 1937, Mrs. E.S. gave birth to a daughter. When the nurse visited her in mid-November, the parents and two children were living in "two very small, dirty rooms above a vacant store building." The mother was not interested in postpartum care and well-baby instruction. "Mother says she has to work very hard. It is necessary for her to carry water from a store across the street as her husband refused to do this," reported the nurse. Fortunately, the baby appeared well. During a revisit in early December, the nurse reported that the home conditions remained poor and the mother's "diet inadequate. Bread, meat, and milk are all she gets to eat. She says if she purchases other foods, her husband scolds her. Patient appears very tired and undernourished."

Although mothers might resist using physicians for antenatal and well-baby care, nurses did not need to convince them to do so in cases of illness. Because her baby was having trouble breathing, Mrs. E.S. had gone to the doctor, who prescribed treatment. The nurse assisted by demonstrating the proper method of applying nose drops, but she could have little effect on the depressing home situation.[29] Most nurses understood the detrimental effects of poverty in the lives of rural mothers, but when they saw extreme cases like these, which they noted were fairly rare, they were disheartened.[30]

Other mothers resisted medical advice for different reasons. Some were confident in their own abilities. One nurse was baffled by Mrs. M.F., who would not accept the importance of medically directed well-baby care. Mrs. M.F.'s succinct rationale: "It is not necessary – all my children are well."[31] In other instances, the opposition of a grandmother, or even a father, thwarted the nurse's influence. An astute nurse could, nevertheless, turn around such situations. Some of the most extensive narrative reports concern just such triumphs. Voge called on a three-week-old infant and mother in far northeastern Wisconsin in June 1942. As soon as she entered the home, the father, "the supreme head of the household," came in from the field. The breastfed baby was nursed whenever hungry, a practice approved by the father. Voge, though, was firmly convinced of the importance of regularity. She "took this opportunity to use the cow in comparison with the mother, by saying, 'Surely you would not take the cow in from the pasture and milk her at any time of the day. As you no doubt know, if you did this, you would find that the cow would lose her milk.' The father replied, 'There you are right, nurse, *absolutely*. That would be true of Mrs. too. I did not think of that, but she is like a cow. It's all a habit and if the baby gets in the regular habit, that's right.'" The father was now interested in what Voge had to say in many other areas of infant care. She left him with a copy of *Infant Care*, which he planned to read and explain to the mother. "In this way he could show authority," Voge explained in her report, noting that at the end of the visit, the father walked with her to the car, thanked her, and invited her to come again.[32] Apparently, this father became an enthusiast for medically directed infant care. He was persuaded by arguments that resonated with his agricultural experiences.

Pragmatic argumentation influenced many rural mothers to turn to the state nurses. Slowly, many mothers learned that in following the nurse's instructions, their children were healthier and their lives were easier. Others turned to nurses for assistance because of frightening past experiences, potential future disasters, and current problems. Whether responding to positive or negative influences, such mothers wholeheartedly embraced increasing medical intervention in their lives and the lives of their children.

The nurses' reports are filled with stories about joyous patients who earnestly adopt medically sanctioned infant care. In relating her 1936 travels through eastern Wisconsin, Cook frequently noted that "patient pleased for talk with nurse" and "patient would like to have nurses keep in touch with her and teach care of infant."[33] Marie Skog wrote of a mother in western Wisconsin who was "pleased with success she is having in training for toilet habits" (this with a four-month-old infant).[34] Although patients would seem "uninterested" during their visits, nurses were gratified to learn that the mothers later followed their instructions.[35] They would glory in writing about acceptance by "hopeless" cases and how much the conditions of health and home had improved.[36]

In describing how nurses tempered their clients' reluctance toward medical supervision, some of the narratives border on hyperbole. In September 1937, a nurse visited Mrs. E.E. in Clayton, a small town in far western Wisconsin. Initially, the thirty-two-year-old mother with eight children "resented" the nurse's intervention. However, "after talking to her a while she changed her attitude and asked about feeding her baby and how much water to give him. She also promised to start cod liver oil and orange juice at the time the baby is three weeks old."[37]

What could the nurse have said to convince a mother of eight to change her infant care practices? Or, is it possible that Mrs. E.E. simply saw agreement as the easiest way to get the nurse to leave? Alice Rude faced that question in central Wisconsin a few years later. Mothers would agree with all her suggestions and then she would see the same problems during her next visit. She could not decide whether the mothers "need a little more supervision at proper intervals, or whether it is wasting time to visit them."[38] Nordley believed that the "threat" of more intense supervision could persuade some mothers to acquiesce to her directions. She was particularly concerned to get prenatal patients to visit the doctor early in their pregnancies. Not all her clients were eager to do so, but they went. Nordley concluded, "Some of them are a little reluctant about going but perhaps they will feel they would rather go than to tell me they haven't been there when I call again."[39]

In other instances, mothers basically needed health care professionals to validate their childrearing practices. In Amery, a small town in far western Wisconsin, a nurse found the mother of baby E. "very anxious about her baby, worried that baby is getting along o.k." Because the nurse found a baby who was on a four-hour breast-feeding schedule, who received the appropriate doses of cod liver oil and orange juice, and who seemed in good health, she "advised mother to continue same routine and stop worrying."[40] This is not to say that mothers were passive in the presence of nursing assistance; they did, though, use the nurses as a check on their own sense of appropriate infant care. Convinced of the need for modern medical supervision, mothers then looked to nurses to tell them how to carry out correct practices. Mrs. H was adhering to a three-hour feeding schedule for her one-month-old infant. When she noticed that the baby often slept longer than three hours, she queried the nurse about using a four-hour schedule. This mother obviously had been convinced of the importance of regularity in feeding and also the importance of regular bowel movements because she had been giving her very young child enemas. Endorsing the four-hour schedule and reassuring the mother that "a stool every other day is all right with the breast-fed baby," the nurse suggested prune juice, orange juice, and cod liver oil, rather than an enema.[41]

Although the nurses were sure of their prescriptions, there were times when their recommendations conflicted with those of local physicians. Attempting to appear in agreement with the physician could place a nurse in a quandary: how to give mothers the information the nurse believed was needed and appropriate while not directly contradicting the physician or undermining his position as the medical expert? (Virtually all the physicians I have identified in this study are male; all the nurses are female.) In some instances, nurses endeavored tactfully to persuade mothers of the validity of their philosophy of infant care, rather than that of the doctor. Rude worried because the physicians of Juneau County, in central Wisconsin, did not advise mothers to boil babies' milk, which she considered vital to the health of the infants. So, she "diplomatically told" the women to "scald the milk in a double boiler for a few minutes."[42] In other instances, medical publications played a major role in shaping child care practices. "The situation here is rather difficult," read a report from the village of DeForest, in south-central Wisconsin. The one local physician "tells the mothers that if God intended for the baby to have cod liver oil the baby would be born with a bottle of it in his hand and if He intended for the child to have orange juice God would send a crate for him from Heaven. . . . Despite his advice we found quite a few of the mothers following the Infant Care book and giving the babies cod liver oil and orange juice."[43] Because there was a clear consensus between the nurses' Standing Orders and Children's Bureau pamphlets such as *Infant Care*, a mother was receiving high praise indeed when she was reported to be "following Infant Care."

Conclusion

Confident in their knowledge of infant and child care, the nurses of the Bureau of Maternal and Child Health endeavored to persuade mothers to follow the best medical advice available. In addition to directions for infant feeding, bathing, and toilet training, the modern regime was characterized by the regular involvement of the physician in prenatal, postnatal, and well-baby care. The separation of public health and private medicine – the need to ward off any charge of "state medicine" – necessitated that the state nurses be ever alert to the needs and desires of the local physicians (regardless of whether they agreed with the standards of practice promoted by the nurses and the Bureau) and to ensure that women and their children regularly saw physicians. However, the nurses were also aware that not all physicians agreed with contemporary well-baby care as set forth in *Infant Care*, and that regular physician visits were impossible or impractical for many women in rural Wisconsin because of their economic or geographic situations. The reports of the Wisconsin public health nurses who struggled to improve the lives and health of their rural clients can provide important insights into the ways that gender relations are reproduced and negotiated and how contemporary health care policy, norms of medical practices, and patient circumstances constrain and define the delivery of health care to those in need.

Rima D. Apple, PhD
Professor of Human Ecology
University of Wisconsin–Madison
1300 Linden Drive
Madison, WI 53706

Notes

1. Narrative Report, Mildred Cook, RN, Brown and Kewaunee Counties, October 1936, Wisconsin Bureau of Maternal & Child Health, Programs & Demonstrations, 1922–61 Collection, Wisconsin Historical Society Archives, Madison, Series 2253 (hereafter WBM&CH), Box 11, Folder 11.

2. Narrative Reports of Louise Steffen and Hazel A. Nordley, WBM&CH, Box 11, Folder 10.

3. For more on the impact of federal funding on Wisconsin's rural health projects, see Sean Patrick Adams, "'Who Guards Our Mothers, Who Champions Our Kids?': Amy Louise Hunter and Maternal and Child Health in Wisconsin, 1935–61," *Wisconsin Magazine of History,* 83 (2000): 181–201.

4. Jeffrey P. Brosco, "The Early History of the Infant Mortality Rate in America: A Reflection upon the Past and a Prophecy of the Future," *Pediatrics,* 103, no. 2 (1999): 478–85; Alisa Klaus, *Every Child a Lion: The Origins of Maternal and Infant Health Policy in the United States and France, 1890–1920* (Ithaca, NY: Cornell University Press, 1993); Deborah Dwork, *War Is Good for Babies and Other Young Children: A History of the Infant and Child Welfare Movement in England, 1898–1918* (London: Tavistock, 1987); Jane Lewis, *The Politics of Motherhood: Child and Maternal Welfare in England, 1900–39* (London: Croom Helm, 1980); Seth Koven and Sonya Michel, eds., *Mothers of a New World: Maternalist Politics and the Origins of Welfare States* (New York: Routledge, 1993); Katherine Arnup, *Education for Motherhood: Advice for Mothers in Twentieth-Century Canada* (Toronto: University of Toronto Press, 1994); and Linda Bryder, *Not Just Weighing Babies: Plunket in Auckland, 1908–98* (Auckland: Pyramid Press, 1998).

5. Recently, historians have begun to address the imbalance between urban and rural studies. See, for example, Lynn Curry, "Modernizing the Rural Mother: Gender, Class, and Health Reform in Illinois, 1910–30," in Rima D. Apple and Janet Golden, eds., *Mothers & Motherhood: Readings in American History* (Columbus: The Ohio State University Press, 1997), 495–516; Curry, *Modern Mothers in the Heartland: Gender, Health, and Progress in Illinois, 1900–30* (Columbus: The Ohio State University Press, 1999); and Julia Grant, "Caught Between Common Sense and Science: The Cornell Child Study Clubs, 1925–45," *History of Education Quarterly,* 34, no. 4 (1994): 433–52.

6. For more on the development of the ideology of scientific motherhood, see Rima D. Apple, "Constructing Mothers: Scientific Motherhood in the Nineteenth and Twentieth Centuries," *Social History of Medicine,* 8 (1995): 161–78, and Apple, *Perfect Motherhood: Science and Childrearing in America* (New Brunswick, NJ: Rutgers University Press, 2006).

7. Much of the material for these paragraphs is drawn from Molly Ladd-Taylor, *Mother-Work: Women, Child Welfare, and the State,* 1890–1930 (Urbana: University of Illinois Press, 1994). See also Kriste Lindenmeyer, *"A Right to Childhood": The U.S. Children's Bureau and Child Welfare, 1912–46* (Urbana: University of Illinois Press, 1997).

8. Of course, the staff of the Bureau did do more. As letters flooded in from concerned mothers across the United States, staff members would respond with advice and even with money. They also contacted local agencies to provide additional assistance to mothers in need. Much of this they did from their own resources because the Bureau's finances were always limited and their mandate restricted. For examples of the Bureau's work, see Lindenmeyer, *"A Right to Childhood";* Emily K. Abel, "Correspondence Between Julia C. Lathrop, Chief of the Children's Bureau, and a Working-Class Woman, 1914–15," *Journal of Women's History,* 5, no. 1 (1993): 79–88; and Molly Ladd-Taylor, *Raising a Baby the Government Way: Mothers' Letters to the Children's Bureau, 1915–32* (New Brunswick, NJ: Rutgers University Press, 1986).

9. The Sheppard-Towner Maternity and Infancy Protection Act resulted in part from passage of the women's suffrage amendment and politicians' interest in currying favor with the newly enfranchised women. Also, during World War I, approximately one third of the thousands of men examined for military service were deemed unfit for duty. Medical reports concluded that the defects that led to rejection had their origins in early infancy and with proper care would have never occurred. "Wisconsin's Child Welfare Special: Resumé of Five Years' Work, 1922 to 1926," WBC&MH, Box 16, Folder 1.

10. Health clinics were not new with the Sheppard-Towner Act. Various local governmental and nongovernmental agencies had established semipermanent and traveling clinics in the first two decades of the twentieth century. See, for example, Susan L. Smith, *Sick and Tired of Being Sick and Tired: Black Women's Health Activism in America, 1890–1950* (Philadelphia: University of Pennsylvania Press, 1995) for a discussion of clinics set up by African-American women's clubs.

11. Miss Connor's Case Report [Adams and Waushara Counties], October 23, 1936, WBM&CH, Box 11, Folder 9.

12. Miss Connor's Case Report, 1936.

13. Miss Connor's Case Report, 1936.

14. Narrative Report, Sadie Engesether, RN, Polk-Burnett Counties, June 1937, WBM&CH, Box 13, Folder 8; emphasis in original. Although the state's nurses typically appeared uncomfortable with their Native American clients, most of the report writers tried to be understanding about the effect of living conditions and racism. "Indian mothers often

show great intelligence in the care of their children. If there is neglect of the child, it most often is neglect due to inability to secure proper food, clothing, and housing conditions for the family. The Indian mother trusts her child in the care of the white medicine woman. She often will walk considerable distance to get advice or help," concluded one Health Department writer in 1926.

15. Miss Connor's Case Report, October 31, 1936.

16. Narrative Report, Nathalie Voge, Marinette County, August 1942, WBM&CH, Box 13, Folder 1.

17. Typical Standing Orders for both nurses' home visits and centers were
1. Breast feeding if possible.
2. Regardless of breast or bottle, on a four-hour schedule, omit 2 A.M. feeding as early as possible, omit 10 P.M. feeding at 6 months; on three meals a day between twelve and fifteen months.
3. Regardless of breast or bottle, begin weaning to cup at nine months, complete by ten months. No breast or bottle after one year.
4. Regardless of breast or bottle, dietary supplements of cod liver oil and orange juice. In 1933, these were begun at six weeks; by 1937, by four weeks of age.
5. Bowel training to begin at three months and be completed by six months.
6. Trained for night wetting by two years.

Drawn from typescript, "Points on Which Doctors Should Agree," 1/12/37, and Dr. E.A. Taylor, "Child Health Center: Technique and Standards," WBM&CH, Box 6, Folder 2.

18. Narrative Reports, Hazel Nordley, RN, Forest County, January, February, April 1940, WBM&CH, Box 1, Folder 4.

19. Narrative Report, Demonstration Nurse, Monroe and Jackson Counties, June 1938, WBM&CH, Box 12, Folder 3.

20. Narrative Report, Dr. Ernest Newman, Schofield [Marathon County], April 23, 1940, WBM&CH, Box 8, Folder 4.

21. Narrative Report, Demonstration Nurse, Monroe and Jackson Counties, July 1938, WBM&CH, Box 12, Folder 3. For more on the campaign against flies in this period, see Naomi Rogers, *Dirt and Disease: Polio Before FDR* (New Brunswick, NJ: Rutgers University Press, 1992).

22. Miss Connor's Case Report, 1936 .

23. Narrative Report, Louise Steffen, RN, Barron County, February 1940, WBM&CH, Box 11, Folder 10.

24. Narrative Report, Catherine McLetchie, RN, Shawno County, August 1942, WBM&CH, Box 13, Folder 13.

25. Narrative Report, Hazel A. Nordley, RN, March and May 1943, Box 11, Folder 10.

26. Narrative Report, Ruth Exner, RN, Grant County, July 1940, WBM&CH, Box 12, Folder 5.

27. *From Morning Until Night* (c. 1937) provides a visual record of the nurses' bathing demonstration. This 16-mm silent film, part of the "Judy" series of silent movies, was produced by the University of Wisconsin for the State Department of Health in the 1930s. It was used in infant-care classes at centers, in high schools, and among community groups. The involved step-by-step demonstration begins with the mother scrubbing her hands and arms up to the elbows. Then the mother washes the infant's eyes and ears with

dampened sterile cotton, weighs the infant, washes the infant's face with a wash cloth, soaps the infant on a changing table, places the infant in a basin and rinses her, dries the infant, and then oils her, before dressing her in a light shirt and diaper. A copy of the film is located in the Archives of the Wisconsin Historical Society.

28. Narrative Report, Thelma Burke, RN, Marathon County, March 1939, WBM&CH, Box 12, Folder 17.

29. Narrative Report, Monroe and Jackson Counties, November 1937; Narrative Report, (Miss) Marie Skog, Demonstration Nurse, Monroe and Jackson Counties, December 1937, both WBM&CH, Box 13, Folder 3.

30. For examples of these cases, see Narrative Reports, Hazel A. Nordley, RN, June 1940, January 1941, February 1941, WBM& & CH, Box 12, Folder 4; Narrative Report, Sadie Engesether, RN, February 1937.

31. Narrative Report, Monroe and Jackson Counties, April 1938, April 22, Camp Douglass Route, WBM&CH, Box 13, Folder 3.

32. Narrative Report, Nathalie Voge, June 1942.

33. Narrative Report, Mildred Cook, RN, October 1936.

34. Narrative Report, (Miss) Marie Skog, Demonstration Nurse.

35. See, for example, Narrative Report, Ruth Exner, RN, October 1940.

36. See, for example, Narrative Report, Elizabeth Murrisy, RN, Marathon County, June 1940, WBM&CH, Box 12, Folder 17; Narrative Report, Sadie Engesether, RN, February 1937.

37. Narrative Report, Sadie Engesether, RN, February 1937.

38. Narrative Report, Alice N. Rude, RN, Juneau County, February 1940, WBM&CH, Box 12, Folder 10.

39. Narrative Report, Hazel Nordley, RN, February 1940, WBM&CH, Box 12, Folder 4.

40. Narrative Report, Sadie Engesether, RN, May 1937.

41. Narrative Report, Monroe and Jackson Counties, June 9, 1938, Fairchild, WBM&CH, Box 13, Folder 3.

42. Narrative Report, Alice N. Rude, RN, June 1940.

43. Narrative Report, Dr. Bessie Mae Beach, Dane County, DeForest, WBM&CH, Box 6, Folder 15.

Reweaving a Tapestry of Care: Religion, Nursing, and the Meaning of Hospice, 1945–1978

Joy Buck
University of Pennsylvania School of Nursing

> . . . people who have worked in general and chronic wards do seem to think it is rather epoch-making that every one of our patients looks peaceful, contented, and free from pain, whenever they come round the hospice. I do not pretend for a moment that [it] is my work. . . . Of course, most of the work is just the good nursing.[1]

When British physician Cicely Saunders wrote those words to a colleague, she was in the process of blending the religious roots of hospice with an academic model of clinical research on pain control for terminally ill cancer patients at St. Joseph's Hospice in London. In preparation for building St. Christopher's, a hospice of her own, she wrote a series of letters to physicians in the United States to learn more about how Americans cared for terminally ill cancer patients. In 1963, Saunders made the first of many trips to the United States to visit medical centers and universities across the country and to lecture about the benefits of the "good nursing" and her work at St. Joseph's. Her eloquent descriptions of the hospice philosophy of care resonated with a small but growing cadre of idealistic nurses, clergy, and physicians who believed that medical care for the dying had grown increasingly impersonal and technologically managed. At the time Saunders began her correspondence with the Americans, she did not know that broad economic, social, and cultural changes underway in the United States were creating an environment ripe for reform. Nor could she have foretold how the transatlantic transfer of knowledge, research, and ideals would serve as a catalyst to ignite the American hospice movement.

This article examines transitions in community-based care for the dying before and after the inception of the American hospice movement. Specifically, the early development of modern hospices in Britain and the state of Connecticut (1945–1974) is used as a case study to examine the interplay among religion, nursing, and the modern conceptualization of hospice. Beginning with a discussion of the antecedents of modern hospices, the article explores how these shaped Saunders's conceptualization of hospice as both place and systematic

Nursing History Review 15 (2007): 113–145. A publication of the American Association for the History of Nursing. Copyright © 2007 Springer Publishing Company.

approach to caring for the dying. This is followed by an examination of how and why the transatlantic exchange of knowledge and ideas brought a multidisciplinary group together to advance hospice as a necessary health care reform in the United States and the challenges the group faced as they moved toward integrating hospice into the American medical system.

In reconstructing the history of hospice, I argue that, although the modern hospice concept may have been in sharp contrast to standard medical and nursing care for the dying in some academic medical centers, it was not wholly different from nursing care provided at home and in specialized homes for the dying in both Britain and the United States. Although few of these homes were called hospices, they were critical to the modern conceptualization of hospice as both a place and philosophy of care for the dying.

Previous studies of the American hospice movement typically begin by tracing the word hospice, linking earlier hospices to the creation of modern hospitals, and then quickly move to Cicely Saunders and the founding of the modern hospice movement.[2] As historian Clare Humphreys argues, this preoccupation with the term "hospice" has resulted in the obfuscation of the role that other earlier homes for the dying played in caring for the terminally ill.[3] Moreover, the centrality of medical institutions and physicians in these analyses obscures the significance of the roles of families, nurses, and religious groups in community-based care for the dying and the development of modern hospices. Building on previous scholarship on the institutionalization of life's beginning and end in Canada and home care in the United States,[4] this study illuminates the links between faith traditions, personal ideologies, shifting professional paradigms, culture, and class that remain invisible in much modern scholarship of hospice.

Weaving a Tapestry of Care: Early Homes for the Dying

The meaning of hospice has changed through history. The earliest hospices were Christian centers where travelers and the poor, sick, and dying could find comfort and respite. During the late nineteenth and early twentieth centuries, care of the dying was primarily within the realm of the family. Although the "deserving poor" who were sick could enter voluntary hospitals for care, institutional biases afforded higher priority to patients with the potential for cure. Once diagnosed as incurable, the dying poor were sent home or to asylums and almshouses to be cared for until they died.[5] Beginning in the late nineteenth century, a number of homes opened in the British Isles and America to provide specialized care for the hopelessly ill poor. Most, although not all, of these homes were founded and operated by Catholic, Methodist, and Anglican religious groups. Although there were denominational differences in their approach to care for the dying, they were united in their dedication to a "social gospel" that called them to serve the poorest of the poor.[6]

One of the earliest institutions with an explicit commitment to care of the dying was founded by the Irish Sisters of Charity in Dublin. Mother Mary Aikenhead, founder of the order in 1816, had a special love and concern for dying patients that she "honored as pilgrims departing on a longer journey."[7] In 1879, twenty-one years after Mother Aikenhead's death, the sisters founded Our Lady's Hospice, the first hospice in Dublin committed solely to care of the dying. The hospice's initial charter attests to its mission: "Long and sadly has been felt the want of an institution into which those who have no relative or friend to watch beside them in their last hours may be received, tended by charitable hands, comforted and prepared for their passage to eternity."[8]

The sisters soon acquired a reputation for making the "passage from life to death through a brief darkness a happy one." Our Lady's Hospice's first annual report, published in 1882, documented that during its first three years of existence, the nuns provided terminal nursing care for 336 patients and were "generally well received by the public." The report, which was distributed to the hospice's benefactors, characterized the sisters' attitudes toward their patients by the following: "No words can express the gratitude felt by those whose privilege it is to carry out this great work."[9]

Historically, compassion, comfort measures, and spiritual care for the sick and dying were the cornerstones of hospice care. The medical knowledge and technology that make optimal symptom management a possibility today were limited. According to a report of expenditures at the forty-bed Our Lady's Hospice, from September 1881 to September 1882, £518 was spent on meat; £251 on groceries, wine, and spirits; and £175 on medical attendance and pharmacy. The majority of patients at the hospice died of consumption; the mainstay of symptom management was the use of whiskey mixed with milk, a common treatment for many diseases at the time, but especially tuberculosis.[10] The amount spent on the chapel and chaplains was almost identical to that spent on medical attendance and pharmacy and is indicative of the limited pharmacopoeia and the high value early hospices placed on spiritual care for the dying.

At the turn of the twentieth century, the nuns opened another home, St. Joseph's Hospice for the Dying, to meet the medical, social, and religious needs of the terminally ill in London. At St. Joseph's, special attention was given to helping patients achieve what was called "soul cures" when a physical cure was not possible.[11] These "soul cures" depended on the individual's acceptance of the Catholic faith and participation in its specific rituals. Although spiritual healing was paramount, it was generally accepted that this could not be accomplished until the person's physical and mental suffering had been alleviated. The individual was the primary focus of care, but a patient's social and familial relationships were also important. "The sisters believed that happy and holy deaths should be edifying to others, especially non-Catholic relatives, and that estranged family members should be reconciled."[12] Thus, care was extended to the patients' families as well.

Another example of an early home for the terminally ill in London was St. Luke's Home for the Dying Poor, founded in 1893 by Dr. Howard Barrett, with affiliations with the Methodist Church.[13] Like St. Joseph's, St. Luke's made clear distinctions between paupers and the "respectable poor" the institution was meant to serve.[14] Whereas the power and authoritative control of St. Joseph's was vested in the Mother Rectress, at St. Luke's it was vested in the medical director.[15] St. Luke's was thus under secular management and staffed by lay nurses, yet the influence of Methodist theology was evident in the approach to dying. As at St. Joseph's, religious faith was a critical component of care. The Methodists believed, however, that the dying person's "faith in Jesus" within the broader context of Christianity was more important than religious conversion to a particular denomination.[16] The hospice staff were duty bound by their charter to respect the "absolute sanctity" of the individual and to "try to reach that which makes the man *himself*, and does not belong to another."[17] Barrett attested to this philosophical approach in a 1909 report: "We do not think or speak of our inmates as 'cases.' We realize that each one is a human microcosm, with its own characteristics, its own life history, intensely interesting to itself and some small surrounding circle."[18] As such, each individual's personal characteristics and history were incorporated into the care he or she received.

In the United States as in Britain, there were many groups dedicated to service to the dying poor. One of these, the Servants for the Relief of Incurable Cancer, was a tertiary Dominican nursing order founded by Rose Hawthorne Lathrop and Alice Huber.[19] Lathrop began her work after training as a nurse at the New York Cancer Hospital during the summer of 1896.[20] Initially, she visited patients in their homes, dressed their wounds, and provided what services she could to family members. She was soon joined by Huber, and in 1899, they were accepted into the Dominican Third Order and opened St. Rose's Free Home for Incurable Cancer in New York City.[21] At St. Rose's, careful attention was given to making the rooms look bright, cheerful, and homelike. In the summer, patients who were able to move about could sit and walk in a small yard filled with plants. Patients were welcomed regardless of religion, race, ethnicity, or condition of poverty. No class distinctions were made between "deserving" and "nondeserving" poor, and no money was accepted for the services provided.

Although the Dominican habits the sisters wore evidenced their religious faith, proselytizing was strictly prohibited. No one was allowed to "show abhorrence or disgust at the sight of repulsive ugliness brought about by cancer."[22]

A prolific writer, Lathrop deplored the use of terminally ill patients for medical research and often wrote of her disdain in newspaper and magazine articles, correspondence, and in *Christ's Poor*, a small magazine intended to inform an ever-widening group of benefactors of their work.[23] For example, when one patient came to the home after discharge from a local hospital with almost half of her face "eaten away" by cancer, Lathrop wrote: "I suppose she is one of those whom they publish that they can 'cure.' I wish someone would stop those unstinted lies about cure which even that good hospital stoops to printing – for the sake of attracting subjects for experiment."[24] In contrast, the sisters eased the patient's suffering through morphine, fresh air, and "whatever dainties the patients desired." They were duty bound by the group's covenants to assure that patients, once deemed incurable, were not used as guinea pigs for medical research.[25] Lathrop did not believe, as most did, that cancer was contagious, and she called on nurses to overcome their fears and provide much needed care for the cancerous poor.

She kept meticulous notes and wrote to a benefactor of her desire to publish her findings:

> I've been thinking this morning what a lot of valuable information we have collected during all these years of work. How best to relieve pain for the hopelessly sick; how to help do away with the odor of cancer. You see that patients feel terribly about that, and it upsets their nerves and so makes their physical condition worse. And I'd like to tell them how some dressings and some treatments are literally worse than none, for they aggravate the condition rather than helping it. And I'd tell them how cheerfulness toward these patients is almost the best treatment of all.[26]

Unfortunately, she died soon after this letter was written. Her wish to further disseminate this valuable information was never realized.

In this brief examination of early homes for the dying, one can note several cornerstones of the modern hospice philosophy and practice. They all had altruistic missions, were united by their commitment to care for the dying, and were respectful of the patient's individuality. Despite denominational differences in the approach to dying and management of the deathbed, the patient was universally perceived as being composed of three distinct yet interrelated entities: mind, body, and soul. The alleviation of physical and emotional symptoms was considered a prerequisite to healing the soul. Although optimal management of physical symptoms was restricted somewhat by the limited pharmacopoeia of the day, all means available were used to alleviate the patients' suffering.

Special attention was given to creating a place that was welcoming, homelike, and comforting. The hospices emphasized the importance of "being with" patients through their final hours and attended to their individual needs. Although there was not an explicit commitment to care for the family, there was concern over the patients' social context, in general, and the family, in particular.

Despite the prevalence of these antecedents of modern hospices, the value of the care they provided has not been widely appreciated. Yet, they are directly linked to the modern hospice movement by Cicely Saunders, who worked at St. Joseph's and St. Luke's as a nurse, medical almoner (social worker), and finally physician. Both homes played a critical role in her beliefs and approach to care for the dying on which the modern conceptualization of hospice would be built.

Cicely Saunders and the Conceptualization of an Ideal

Although Saunders began her career in health care as a nurse in 1940, she was soon "invalided" by a back injury. Desiring to stay in the medical field, she then trained as a medical almoner (social worker). While working in this capacity at St. Luke's Home, her commitment to improving care for terminally ill cancer patients began. It was there in 1947 that she met David Tasma, a forty-year-old agnostic Polish Jewish refugee who was dying of cancer. During their short but emotionally intense relationship, Saunders's dream to open a home for the dying began to take shape. As Tasma's death drew near, they discussed the needs of dying patients and how best to meet them. Although Saunders wanted Tasma to be converted to Christianity before he died, she respected his religious viewpoint and his need to walk his own path. Before Tasma died, he willed Saunders £500, saying "I'll be a window in your home."[27] It would be nineteen years before that home, St. Christopher's Hospice, became a reality in London.

Within several days of Tasma's death, Saunders volunteered her services as a nurse at St. Luke's Home for the Dying. In this capacity, she was introduced to a unique concoction of medications and alcohol used in the management of pain, the Brompton Cocktail.[28] The use of this mixture had been initiated at the home during the early 1930s, but its use and benefits were not widely known in medical circles. More important to the drug's effectiveness was the novel method of delivering medication. It was given orally rather than by injection, and it was given on a routine basis rather than requiring the patient to ask for it. This practice was based on experience and the premise that once patients were allowed to feel pain, it took more time and greater dosages of medication to alleviate it. The belief that preventing pain by around-the-clock dosing was preferable to treating existing pain would become central to Saunders's care of the dying: controlling pain before it controlled the patient.[29] Also central to her future care of the dying was the use of a combination of medications, or "polypharmacy," to manage multiple symptoms.

By the mid-1950s, Saunders was solidly committed to care of the dying and sought to return to nursing full time. A thoracic surgeon and mentor from St. Thomas's recommended that, rather than return to nursing, she should "go and read medicine. It's the doctors who desert the dying."[30] Although Saunders loved bedside nursing, based on her observations of Dr. Barrett at St. Luke's Hospice, she concurred that medical training was in all likelihood necessary to gain the requisite power and authority to direct and improve medical management of terminally ill cancer patients.

By the time Saunders finished her medical training, rapid advances in pharmacotherapy had significantly increased the numbers and quality of drugs available for pain and symptom management. New synthetic narcotics and other drugs, such as new psychotropics, phenothiazines, antidepressants, anxiolytics, synthetic steroids, and nonsteroidal anti-inflammatory drugs, offered tools to ameliorate a wide range of symptoms, but their efficacy in the management of terminal disease had yet to be empirically tested. Armed with a clinical research fellowship from the Department of Pharmacology at St. Mary's Hospital Medical School, Saunders approached the Irish Sisters of Charity with a proposal to work at St. Joseph's Hospice and conduct clinical research on patients' terminal pain and its relief. While there, Saunders's research resonated with the young house staff physicians, and they became her disciples in legitimizing palliative symptom management for the terminally ill through clinical research. The findings from their ongoing research served as ammunition in the fight for effective pharmacological intervention to alleviate suffering, a controversial notion whose time, Saunders believed, had come.[31] It would, however, meet significant opposition from the medical profession.[32]

Although the research was necessary to validate her approach to pain management, Saunders heart was really in patient care. She admired how the sisters at St. Joseph's remained at the bedside to sit with and listen to patients.[33] She wrote of how the sisters' integration of care to mind, body, and soul "transformed the wards."[34] Their approach became central to her evolving understanding of care that focused on "being with" versus "doing to" and placed the needs of the patients and their families at the center of care. Of her time at St. Joseph's Hospice, Saunders wrote: "It soon became clear that each death was as individual as the life that preceded it and that the whole experience of that life was reflected in a patient's dying. This led to the concept of 'total pain,' which is presented as a complex of physical, emotional, social, and spiritual elements. The whole experience for a patient includes anxiety, depression, and fear; concern for the family who will become bereaved; and often a need to find some meaning in the situation, some deeper reality in which to trust."[35]

Building on what she learned at St. Joseph's, Saunders envisioned St. Christopher's, the hospice she hoped to build, as "a community [where] people shared the cost of being vulnerable."[36] She embraced the belief that the dying have intrinsic value and are not inanimate receivers but rather active participants in their care. This philosophy broke down the artificial barriers between the various aspects of care and blurred the boundaries of how health professionals and patients existed in relationship to each other. A charismatic leader and extremely successful at articulating the value of such care, Saunders soon became a powerful force in terminal-care reform.

Hands Across the Waters: Conception of the Modern Hospice Movement

In 1963, Saunders made the first of several trips to the United States and Canada to gain support for St. Christopher's and to learn about the care of terminally ill cancer patients in North America.[37] During an eight-week period, she visited eighteen different hospitals and gave a series of lectures about her work at St. Joseph's. Throughout her U.S. trip, Saunders kept a detailed record of people she met, places she went, and impressions of them. On her return to London, she summarized her recorded observations and what she considered to be the strengths and weaknesses of terminal care in America.[38] The major factors she discussed were (1) physiological pain and symptom management; (2) emotional pain and distress of patients and families; (3) the work of social workers with patients and families; (4) nursing education, research, and writing; (5) chaplain training and work; (6) specialized homes for patients with terminal care; and (7) volunteer programs. Her report was then sent to key people she met while in the United States.[39] Her observations and evaluations indicate that the transfer of knowledge and ideas flowed in both directions, with Americans learning from Saunders and her from them.

From correspondence with several physicians prior to her visit, Saunders knew that there were serious inadequacies in the prevailing models of care for the dying in the United States. Although she assumed that there were no homes for the terminally ill in the United States, she soon learned that she was mistaken. Although finding the homes was not easy, she visited three homes for the dying, all run by religious orders and all in New York. Two of these homes, St. Rose's Home and Rosary Hill, were operated by the Hawthorne Dominicans. By the time of Saunders's 1963 visit, the order that Lathrop and Huber founded ran seven homes for the dying in six states, with a total capacity of 700 beds.[40] Saunders noted that St. Rose's held approximately a hundred beds, arranged in eight- and four-bed wards with few private rooms. The atmosphere was "friendly and homelike with patient pictures and belongings in the right sort of untidiness in the wards."[41] Sixteen nuns, few of whom were trained nurses, provided all of the care with the assistance of one male orderly and a porter. At Rosary Hill Home, also operated by the Hawthorne Dominicans, Saunders found that patients not yet in the terminal phases of their disease often helped care for patients who were. Thus, despite their illness, they contributed to the care of those whose needs were greater than their own. It is interesting to note that, despite the limited training of the care providers, the patients were well cared for.[42]

Due to limitations in time and funding, Saunders did not have opportunity to visit additional homes and institutions committed to the terminally ill.[43] The relative public invisibility of the valuable services provided in these homes reflected not only the humility of the religious orders that ran them but also the curative biases of larger medical institutions, the stigmatization associated with "incurability," and marginalization of care for the dying.

Throughout Saunders's report, her religious conviction, presuppositions about what she would find, and her firm belief in her approach to terminal care and the role of nursing within that were evident. Of nurses, Saunders wrote that many of the trained (professional) nurses were relegated to administrative duties, leaving much of the direct patient care to practical nurses and "aid[e]s."[44] She observed that due to their administrative function, nurses were not involved with patient care, and thus, she reasoned, not fully cognizant of their needs or those of their families.[45] For example, of a British nurse working in Boston, Saunders wrote: "I met a 'head nurse' from Guy's [Hospital in London] . . . [who told me] that the administration and paper work [in the U.S.] were more swamping than in England. She had managed to re-organize her work with the help of a ward secretary and said that at last she was getting near her patients. Nearly all the nursing stations I saw were very well laid out and equipped. But they were usually full of nurses, and, incidentally, that is where I found her too."[46] Saunders also observed that patients often felt "safest with the nurses who are cheerful and ordinary, who can express the feelings spontaneously and share mundane comments on life in and out of the ward."[47] She found the migration of nursing education from training schools to the university a bit "strange to those of us with a practical approach."[48] These comments exposed not only her biases of the appropriate role and function of nurses but also the formalization of the nurse-patient relationship and the creation of a therapeutic milieu.[49]

Regardless of her opinion about the appropriate role, function, and education of nurses, Saunders was complimentary of the nursing education programs she visited. She noted that these programs focused attention on students' understanding of the patient's individual personality, concern with emotional problems, and a "relationship versus task" approach to nursing.[50] As such, she found that the American nurses used a patient-centered approach to care similar to the approach she so admired in the nuns at St. Joseph's. Although she was somewhat critical of the limitations of nursing care for the dying, primarily related to the limited contact "trained nurses had with patients," Saunders believed that the American nurses were quite aware of the inadequacies of the system of care for the dying and were using "much imagination in trying to improve matters." She was also impressed that nurses were involved in several interesting research projects as coinvestigators, assistants, and, in some cases, the principal investigator.[51] She concluded the report by discussing several "valuable exchanges going on today between workers in medicine and nursing and the writers of philosophy and theology."[52] She emphasized the similarities between her work and that of her colleagues in the United States and reflected that on both sides of the Atlantic, many health care professionals and clergy possessed "compassionate simplicity."[53]

"The Moment of Truth": Birth of the American Hospice Movement

Saunders's first trip to the United States marked a pivotal point in terminal-care reform. For one American nurse, Florence Wald, Saunders's 1963 talk to the Yale University School of Nursing proved to be providential.[54] Considered by many to be the "mother of hospice nursing" in the United States, when Wald first heard Saunders speak, she was at a critical point in her life.[55] As dean of the School of Nursing, Wald became a leading advocate for major reforms in nursing education and the clinical role of the nurse.[56] Like Saunders, she believed that professional nurses should "rid themselves" of nonnursing tasks such as "administering the ward, transcribing information, and ordering, giving, and charging drugs" so they might return to the bedside to provide patient care.[57] She had grown increasingly dismayed by the growing trend in medicine to focus on cure and technology rather than on people.[58] Frustrated clinical faculty and students often complained to Wald about physicians who refused to respond to patients' queries such as, "What's wrong with me?" and "Am I going to get better?" When the nurses suggested that they might speak to the patients if the physicians were uncomfortable, they were met with: "If you're going to talk about this, I'm going to see that you're not allowed to see the patient anymore."[59] Based on the research and writing of nursing leaders such as Doris Schwartz and Jean Quint [Benoliel], as well as her observations, Wald believed that communication barriers between patients and professionals were pervasive. Moreover, the "inadequate and ineffective" communication patterns also existed among the professionals. "Both professions [nursing and medicine] bear a responsibility to identify and resolve the conflicts that occasionally arise between them, instead of mutually withdrawing, as often happens today, or one profession deprecating the other."[60] She firmly believed that nurses were able to create the bridge between the seemingly antithetical systems of cure and care and that nurses should be equal partners, including serving as leaders, of interdisciplinary care teams.[61] Saunders's approach encapsulated Wald's thinking about the type of care patients should have across their lifespan. Moreover, the centrality of nursing and the multidisciplinary nature of hospice care was exactly the framework Wald believed was necessary to engender change.

During the next several years, Wald and Saunders maintained correspondence and made plans for Saunders to return as a visiting professor in nursing. Saunders agreed that such a visit would be extremely valuable for her thinking and planning for the future. She also emphasized the importance of clinical training versus theoretical discussions and lectures on palliative symptom management.[62] In 1966, Saunders returned for six weeks as Annie Goodrich Visiting Professor of Nursing. She taught student nurses and made rounds with surgeons, pediatricians, and psychiatrists.[63] In addition, Wald organized two major functions: the Annie Goodrich Visiting Professor Lecture and an Institute on Care of the Terminally Ill. The lecture was held on April 26, and local dignitaries, faculty, students, and hospital staff were invited to attend. The institute was held just prior to Saunders's departure in May.

Saunders's title for the Goodrich lecture, "The Moment of Truth," reflected her understanding that many health professionals felt inadequate in their communications with terminally ill patients and their families.[64] As she introduced the lecture, she emphasized the universality of death and connected it to living: "I have chosen the title 'The Moment of Truth' not because I just want to discuss the perennial questions, 'Should you tell the dying patient the truth?' (which is not the right question anyway), but because meeting dying patients and facing the fact of death does concern all of us, whether we're nurses, doctors, social workers, psychologists, or any other discipline. I think perhaps almost most of all, when we're members of the family."[65] To Saunders, the "moment of truth" involved much more than the logistics of who should say what and when to say it. Rather, the moment had "deep and far-reaching implications" that held relevance to "the whole of life" of humans. To illustrate the benefits to her approach to care for the dying, she shared stories of dying patients who arrived at St. Joseph's expressing feelings of guilt, failure, and rejection. She showed slides of these patients at admission looking anxious and in pain and again during the last days of their lives looking comfortable, alert, and active. These images highlighted the key components of hospice care and captured the good that can come from care that focuses on the alleviation of physical symptoms, as well as the social, psychological, and spiritual dimensions of suffering.[66] As Saunders explained, because St. Joseph's was supported by the Catholic Church and philanthropy, and thus financially independent of the British National Health Service, the care it provided was based on the needs of patients and their families rather than on their ability to pay. As a result, patients and families were comforted that the hospice beds "did not have a kind of parking meter beside them."[67] The notion that they would have a bed as long as they needed it was particularly reassuring to dying patients, who were discharged from acute care hospitals once they were deemed incurable.

Saunders also reflected on the experience of caring for the terminally ill from the perspective of professional and family caregivers. She explained that neither family nor health professionals wanted to see a loved one or patient "swamped with distress caused by the treatment or with drugs" or suffering from a sense of being isolated because people avoided them. Rather, both family and professionals wanted to see someone who was able to be him- or herself. Although many professionals dismissed care for the terminally ill by saying "there is nothing more to be done," Saunders advocated for health professionals to provide care that was relevant to the patients' condition, regardless of curative potential. She stressed that the place and presence were important components of this care. Although Saunders believed "home was the best place," social circumstances often precluded patients from remaining there. Saunders told a story about a patient that illustrated how creating an environment that allowed patients to "be themselves" was a gift to both the dying and the bereaved. When the patient and his wife first entered St. Joseph's, they were both tense; he because he was in pain and she because she felt guilty that she would not be able to care for him until the end. The matron and medical officer welcomed them into the hospice, making them feel at home. His pain was quickly controlled by an analgesic mixture and, in Saunders's words, "He was lying back in his bed filling in his football pools, an English form of gambling. This is really the way to help her; I couldn't take away the parting, but at least she could remember him like this."[68]

Saunders's visit culminated with an Institute on Care of the Terminally Ill. The institute brought together a multidisciplinary group of eminent thinkers and practitioners to exchange information about death, dying, and bereavement. The majority of the approximately thirty people who attended the forum concurred that there were significant deficiencies in the existing models of terminal care in America. The evolving philosophy of hospice care that Saunders described provided an intellectual opportunity for scholars and clinicians to work to further develop hospice as an alternative to dying in an intensely curative medical milieu. Hospice was both a clinical model of care that could be empirically tested and a facility that was amenable to environmental engineering. As such, hospice was invaluable to their collective commitment to terminal-care reform. During the next few years, correspondence among Saunders, Wald, and leaders in the emerging discipline of thanatology proliferated. The free exchange of ideas and research created a connectedness and synergy between them that transcended professional disciplines and geography, and thus the foundation for the modern hospice movement was laid.

St. Christopher's in the Field

Between 1966 and 1968, Wald moved steadily toward her dream of providing hospice care in Connecticut. She maintained correspondence with Saunders and visited St. Christopher's while it was being built. Wald, already immersed in the terminal-care reform literature, contacted another nurse researcher, Jeanne Quint (Benoliel), as well as other leaders of the death-and-dying movement, such as Kübler-Ross.[69] She also discovered an ongoing research study being done at Yale–New Haven Hospital by sociologist August Hollingshead and pediatrician Ray Duff, funded by the U.S. Public Health Service Division of Nursing. The study's findings, published in 1968 in *Sickness and Society*, challenged those who praised medical and technological advances that extended life without a full appreciation of the problems some of these treatments created for patients and their families.[70] These studies documented the need for reform and were invaluable to Wald as she built a case for terminal-care reform in Connecticut.

After stepping down as dean in 1968, Wald took a sabbatical and traveled to England for a working vacation at St. Christopher's after its opening. As she worked on the wards, she experienced firsthand the healing nature of hospice care that Saunders had spoken of so eloquently. This type of nursing resonated to the core of Wald's being, and she returned home with a renewed commitment to hospice that bordered on religious zeal. She wrote to Saunders about her plans to transplant hospice on American soil:

> Cicely, I find it so difficult to thank you – I always do – because you give so abundantly and I know [that] you don't need thanks. Just let me tell you – my three short weeks at St. Christopher's were among the most exquisite of my life. I relive them constantly – not just every day but many times every day. I am so grateful to have been fortunate enough to meet you and everyone whose breath, whose life is St. Christopher's. I only hope that I can be a part of the whole idea and spirit. Now as for what I call 'St. Christopher's in the Field.' My primary effort has been to describe St. Christopher's Hospice. I've begun with family and with friends and then with 'simpatico colleagues.'[71]

The simpatico colleagues she referred to included the Reverend Edward Dobihal, an evangelical Methodist minister with a background in psychotherapy and bereavement, and Morris Wessel, a pediatrician. During the next year, the growing group worked on a plan for a research study on dying patients and their families in the New Haven area. In 1969, they began the "Nurse's Study of the Dying Patient and His Family" with funding from the U.S. Public Health Service Division of Nursing. By August 1970, the research group had grown to include another nurse, Kathy Klaus, and breast-cancer surgeon Ira Goldenberg, and they had gathered enough data to move forward with their plans to build "St. Christopher's in the Field."

On October 29, 1970, the group met to formalize plans with Saunders and Sister McNulty, a nurse and matron at St. Christopher's, in attendance. McNulty accompanied Saunders on the 1970 trip to learn more about clinical research at several American nursing schools. In the meeting, the group outlined issues for consideration and a road map of how to proceed.[72] Beginning with purpose and philosophy, Saunders started the discussion by describing St. Christopher's. She emphasized the religious foundation the hospice was built on but stressed that it was nondenominational and the importance for professionals and patients to be able to define religion in their own terms.[73] The group then shared their individual thoughts and motivation for moving forward with the hospice. Goldenberg, an observant Jew, believed that there was a need in the community to "minister to" terminally ill patients in need. "We are here to set up a facility that will meet a need in the community."[74] In response, Saunders provided explicit information on how they handled various situations at St. Christopher's.

Soon after this meeting, Dobihal traveled to St. Christopher's. Both he and his wife Shirley, a licensed practical nurse, worked on the wards and attended meetings for seven months. They found St. Christopher's to be a unique institution for learning and teaching, and their prolonged stay afforded them the opportunity to fully engage in the work there. St. Christopher's environment was in sharp contrast to the American teaching hospitals, both in its approach to patients and their families and in the professionals' approach to each other.[75] Once admitted to the hospice, patients were welcomed by the matron and medical officer, made to feel at home, and reassured that their bed would be theirs for as long as they needed it. Hospice personnel were mutually supportive and shared responsibility for the "total work of the hospice."[76] The interdisciplinary senior staff, which included Saunders, the director of nursing, and other administrative heads, met on a weekly basis, as did the nursing staff. A larger interdisciplinary group met on a biweekly basis to discuss specific issues such as research and financial matters. Smaller groups also met on a weekly basis to discuss a series of philosophical topics, such as the meaning of "being a person" and "freedom." These small-group discussions were attended by a diverse gathering of professionals, staff, and volunteers. As important to Dobihal, prayer groups were held three times a day in the chapel and led by various members of the staff.[77]

Dobihal was pleased to learn that this religious framework was not distasteful to Jewish and agnostic patients. To the contrary, he found that they respected it and "spoke positively about the religious practices even if they chose not to participate in services." This was important to him for several reasons. First, there were several people on the research team who were uncomfortable with the overtly Christian foundations of St. Christopher's. Like Saunders, Dobihal saw hospice care as an extension of faith. Frustrated by the prevailing medical institution's bias toward care of the temporal body to the exclusion of psychological and spiritual realms, he was convinced that the American hospice must have a religious base that was equal to the medical.[78]

While Dobihal was in England, Wald continued her efforts to garner support for hospice. Upon his return to the United States, the group was ready to "shift gears" and quicken the pace toward its goal of building a hospice.[79] They decided to split the growing group of supporters into two subgroups. A steering committee was created comprising the research team, Lutheran minister Frederick Auman, and Catholic priest Robert Canny. Social psychologist Sherry Israel was invited to serve as a process recorder to observe and document the group's collective dynamics.[80] They met on a weekly basis and bore primary responsibility for the hospice's planning and development. The second, larger group was composed of a growing group of hospice supporters who would help with various task forces. They also met on a weekly basis, and Dobihal served as chair of both groups.[81]

Between March and May 1971, the steering committee discussed many topics. The group expended a considerable amount of time and energy developing a statement of philosophy and underlying assumptions about hospice care. Although they used St. Christopher's as their model, for a variety of reasons, their hospice would have a distinctly American flair. The group quickly agreed on three assumptions. First, hospice was a "total community" that included staff, patients, their families, their social context, and the community at large. Within this context, care would be directed by the expressed desires of patient and family about how "they wished to be served." Second, the hospice facility would be physically structured to maximize socialization and community participation. Unlike St. Christopher's "open ward," adaptations in the environmental design would be made to accommodate the "American routine and expectations" for privacy and autonomy. Third, the group would use aninterdisciplinary approach to their work. Professional roles would be blurred to allow professionals to "substitute" for each other and "call on each other for help."[82]

A fourth assumption, concerning the role of religion, resulted in a debate over whether the religious underpinning of hospice care should be implicit or explicit. Saunders planned the creation of St. Christopher's with a lay group and cautioned the American group that if clergy were involved, it was important not to build them or their religious views into the development of the hospice.[83] This view may well have been due to her desire to emulate the St. Luke's Hospice model, which had a medical director and a Christian base. It also reflected her desire to maintain control over St. Christopher's without interference from others. St. Christopher's had both a medical and a religious component; medicine was essential, but religion was an explicit element of care. Saunders identified certain acts, such as nursing care, as religious acts. In a semiecumenical approach, she embraced Christianity rather than a specific religious orthodoxy within it as the central element of care. She described St. Christopher's as having a "Christian base" rather than a "religious" one.[84]

Whether Christian or religious in nature, the question of how to integrate this spiritual component of care was vexing to the American group for two primary reasons: their perceptions of the federal government's grant requirements for the separation of church and state, and the demographics of the religiously plural steering committee. The group struggled to find the proper language that would accommodate myriad faiths and personal philosophies. Dobihal and other clergy on the steering committee wanted those who used "religious vocabulary" to feel at home using it at the hospice, rather than having to "translate everything into secular language."[85] As they discussed the use of the word "God" in their philosophy statement, there were some who believed it was a universal term with which everyone could identify. To others, the group was united by the collective sense of "goodness," and the unifying element was their working toward a common goal rather than religious orthodoxy. Within this context, they believed humanism rather than religion was the common denominator among people and served as the basis of all religions and sects.[86]

This debate over the explicit and implicit foundation of hospice provides interesting insight into the two groups' views of nursing. Saunders believed nursing was at the core of hospice, although she also thought it should be under the direction of a physician. Because nurses were omnipresent and responsible for blending various approaches in the care of patients and their families, she and Wald were in agreement that the hospice was essentially synonymous with nursing. As such, hospice was a nursing facility. Within that context, the chaplain would be brought in when necessary as a "religious consultant," much like the role of the physician and social worker who each had their own niche and who made recommendations about care as consultants.[87]

After several months, the group agreed on a philosophy statement that reflected their collective idealistic fervor, their commitment to hospice, and their struggle for an inclusive philosophy:

> Our philosophy cannot be a creed and yet our explorations and growing bonds cause us to often say, 'We believe.' We believe in honoring the creed and philosophy of every man. We believe in the dignity of personhood – patients, families, workers – and will nurture a spirit of respect of every person. We believe in the importance of feelings, in the fact that there are differences between people to be creatively shared, in love which can be experienced between people and will support them. Some say 'We believe in God' in different ways, but important in that our daily work reflects a purpose that is beyond us and is moving us. . . . This philosophy cannot be concluded in words, for it is one to be tested in action, to remain open to the learning that will come from our relationships with each other, and to be creatively changed and added to.[88]

Despite their idealistic statement of philosophy, the group was cognizant of more pragmatic issues such as funding, organization, and structure. One of their primary concerns was whether they should have a fiscal intermediary, such as a hospital or university, or whether they should serve as their own agent. In part, the answer to this question depended on regulatory and financing mechanisms at the state and federal levels, something they knew little about.

Between 1971 and 1974, a loosely defined group of idealists created a non-profit corporation, Hospice, Inc., and were well on their way to making their dream of St. Christopher's in the Field a reality. As new board members and staff came on board, they traveled to England to experience St. Christopher's firsthand. They returned home with a slightly different interpretation of how the hospice philosophy should be translated into the American medical system. During these formative years, the hospice advocates received a valuable lesson on the difficulties they faced in navigating the Connecticut medical system and gaining community and political support for hospice. Although Saunders continued to be an important influence on the group, they would need to re-create and clearly articulate their own vision of hospice in terms that were palatable to a broad base of individuals and institutions. For example, although not explicitly stated, hospice's focus on "helping people die well" was inconsistent with the curative nature of the medical mainstream. The media had published stories about St. Christopher's and the use of experimental and illegal drugs such as LSD and heroin to treat pain and other symptoms of dying.[89] Given the antidrug sentiment and societal discourse on euthanasia, abortion, and patients' rights at this time, the possibility for public and professional backlash against hospice was very real.[90] In addition, unlike Saunders, who chose to remain independent of the National Health Service in England, the group sought integration into the American system early in the planning stages. Moreover, they needed to define hospice as a patient-care model that was "distinctly different from care in nursing homes or hospitals" so they would not be seen as duplicating services or competing with existing programs.[91]

Initially, the group considered incorporating an inpatient hospice unit into an established acute-care facility—namely, Yale–New Haven Hospital—but financial concerns and space limitations made this not feasible. They next investigated renovation of a nearby convalescent home but decided that this facility was too large for their purposes and the cost of reconstruction would be more than construction of a new facility. With the possibilities of moving into existing buildings exhausted, the group decided on new construction. The group hired Yo-Li Chan as their architect, primarily because of his talent, his willingness to travel to St. Christopher's, and the fact that he had never designed a health care facility. Although one would typically look for someone with previous experience with a certain facility type, they did not want their architect "tainted" by preconceptions of what a health care facility should be.[92] Rather, they wanted someone who could make sensitive observations about the needs of patients, families, and care providers and translate these into the architectural design.

While at St. Christopher's, Chan observed that dying patients were often anxious about time; there was "either not enough of it or too much." He also found that beauty and reminders of the continuation of life could be healing for both patients and family. Based on these observations, his design made liberal use of windows and skylights to help patients mark the "natural passage of time, from sunrise to sunset, from season to season."[93] In addition, the building's design incorporated a number of "transition spaces" that served as "escape valves" for patients, family, and staff. The rooms had corridors on either side; one served a utilitarian purpose, and the other opened into a greenhouse large enough to accommodate visits from patients and family, even if they were bedridden. The greenhouse opened to the outdoors, again with doors large enough to accommodate easy access by patients. According to Chan, this attention to space and nature were important to patients and their families: "When life is coming to an end, the idea of being closed in is very frightening, so in every part of the building we tried to create a feeling of openness. Even when the doors of the glassed greenhouse corridor cannot be opened, patients still have a view of the terrace. The plants also help create the feeling of being able to go out, which is very reassuring to patients."[94]

Although the group had developed an esthetically pleasing and purposeful facility design, they still faced a long and hard uphill battle to achieve licensure for it. The hospice they envisioned did not fit neatly into existing health-facility licensing categories. Because of the interdisciplinary nature of hospice and the skill required to assess, diagnose, and treat symptoms, hospice was more than "nursing home care," which many considered to be primarily custodial. Moreover, competition for limited resources within the health care system was keen, and the chairman of the State Hospital Licensing Council was also the president of the State Nursing Home Association. Based on the assumption that hospice would compete for patients, he took a dim view of their certificate-of-need proposal.[95] Stymied in these quarters, they decided to seek designation as a chronic disease hospital, and in August 1973, they received an endorsement for forty-four chronic-disease beds, with two caveats: the facility had to be located in New Haven, Ansonia, or Seymour, and the site must be selected and approved within one month.[96] They were unsuccessful in achieving these conditions and moved on to explore other options.

Hospice, Inc., was interested in several properties, but the most promising site was in a residential neighborhood in Hamden. Building a health care facility in a residential area required a change in zoning, which in turn required another public hearing. During the public hearing, a panel of hospice representatives made a compelling and emotional presentation to a standing-room-only crowd. They were unprepared for the response they received from the audience. Several questions, such as, "Isn't it dangerous to have dying patients out where there aren't any intensive care units?" and "Why do you need such a beautiful building, these people are dying, after all?," revealed professional and cultural biases about death and the terminally ill.[97] These questions were relatively benign, but they were accompanied by more vexing questions and comments that compared hospice to euthanasia at best and the methods of the Nazis at worst. Additional questions were related to professional and agency domain and included, "Why do we need hospice when we have nursing homes and hospitals?" and "Doesn't the VNA do this already?" As telling, physicians demanded an answer as to what role they would have in hospice and concerns about turning cancer patients into drug addicts. Their expression of these concerns, in turn, elicited even more hostility among the audience. Although there was some vocal support in the room, the unexpected and heated opposition resulted in a denial of their proposal.[98]

The message was loud and clear. Hospice had been so immersed in their mission that they failed to keep their finger on the pulse of the community. The group had done years of soul-searching and discussion about these issues; many in the community had not. They had not done enough work to educate the public about hospice and garner community support before moving ahead with their plans. Moreover, their idealism and passion were not sufficient to guide them through the politically fraught maze of the Connecticut medical system.[99] It became clear that if the hospice was to succeed, they needed someone who was politically savvy. Dennis Rezendes fit the bill and was retained as a consultant to the board. Rezendes had a BA in public administration and had worked closely with the mayor and New Haven government, as well as on Connecticut governor Ella Grasso's political campaign and transition team. This politically astute consultant possessed the skills, knowledge, and contacts that would help the hospice board deal with regulatory agencies and obtain licensure.[100]

As the group moved forward, they learned from their mistakes and carefully honed their message to emphasize the positive aspects of hospice and mitigate the negative. They received funding from a variety of private foundations and local and state governments for facility planning, community education, and home-care-program development. Each proposal the group submitted reflected the ongoing refinement of the hospice concept of care that would not only offer an alternative to existing models of care for the dying but also approximate the medical model by emphasizing the management of symptoms. Even so, they used the stories of patients and their families to garner support for hospice. For example, the proposal the group submitted for a national hospice demonstration project concluded with an uplifting message from Dobihal's experiences at St. Christopher's, a message that was designed to help the reviewers overcome fears related to hospice while demonstrating its need:

In England, I met and talked with patients whose physician had predicted a life expectancy of five to six weeks. I was talking to several of these patients two years later. Their life included work, continuing to maintain the home, gardening, enjoying a holiday, a satisfying personal and social life. The hospice caring for them had not treated their disease but it had loved and cared for them as important persons. One of my dying friends in the hospice in England said, "You know it's **good** to be in this place where I belong, where I felt welcomed. Where people care – even love me. A place where people have time to share with me. They're never too busy for a smile, a word, or to sit down and hold my hand, even cry with me. So you've come all the way from America to learn from us. Well go back and if you don't have places like this, start one for people like me." I heard her request on behalf of others, pray to God daily to help us meet it, and share it now with you.[101]

At the time that Dobihal wrote those words, Hospice, Inc., had more than 200 members, friends, and advisors, including representatives from business, city planning, Blue Cross/Blue Shield and other insurance companies, and Community Health Care Center Plan.[102] With adequate financial resources and their collective broad base of political, professional, and business expertise, a clearly defined mission and plan to achieve it, and hence, emotional appeal, Hospice, Inc., was well positioned to move forward with their home-care program.

Hospice, Inc.: The Modeling of a Movement

Between 1974 and 1980, Hospice, Inc., was transformed from an embryonic home-care program to a projected hospice facility with serious problems to a sustainable program of care for the terminally ill in Connecticut. During this formative period, the hospice philosophy the group espoused was translated into legislation that liberalized reimbursement for home care and officially defined hospice as a special category of chronic-disease hospital. Although Saunders and the Connecticut hospice leaders played a significant role in "spreading the hospice gospel," it was Swiss-born psychiatrist Elisabeth Kübler-Ross who had the most profound impact on the collective consciousness of Americans on the appropriate care for the dying. She helped revolutionize society's conceptualization of death, dying, and bereavement with the publication of her book, *On Death and Dying*, in 1969.[104] Despite her critics, and there were many, Kübler-Ross's writings reached international lay and professional audiences.[106] By the power of her writing and willingness to address the subject of dying, she was able to bridge the academic and grassroots realms of the death-and-dying movements and help stimulate a significant reform of the care of the dying and bereaved.[107] In the early 1970s, nurses commonly cited Kübler-Ross as having the greatest influence on their attitudes toward death, and by 1976, her book had sold more than a million copies.[108] One journalist exclaimed, "No other single person has so dramatically turned around an entire generation of opinion makers on a single subject."[109]

Hospice, Inc., created a National Advisory Council in 1974, with Kübler-Ross as the chair. The primary function of the Council was to transfer information about hospice on two levels: first, to the general public, and second, to hospices across the United States. Through the Council, it was hoped that the public and legislators would become more responsive to the need for the type of care that hospice provided and to "agitate for change in the present health-care delivery system, by reform in the existing institutions and by replication of New Haven's Hospice in their own communities."[110] By 1978, the term "hospice" had been copyrighted and strict criteria were set for its use. Connecticut hospice leaders joined forces with hospice advocates from Florida and other states to form the National Hospice Organization as a mechanism to catapult hospice onto the legislative agenda for Medicare reform.[111]

In 1978, when the author of a *Washington Post* article questioned, "Can the hospice movement take hold in America?," Hospice, Inc., was providing guidance to some hundred local hospice groups across the country.[112] Like Hospice, Inc., many of these fledgling hospices were founded by idealistic nurses, clergy, and physicians. The majority of these hospices started as voluntary efforts and relied heavily on volunteer nurses, often providing patient care, bereavement counseling, and other valuable services after completing their regular shift at work.[113] Others became administrators, community activists, educators, and researchers. With their help, hospice was well on the way to becoming a national phenomenon as a specialized and codified model of care for the terminally ill.

Reweaving the Hospice Tapestry: Lessons from the Past

Throughout much of recent history, society has been hindered in efforts to improve the experiences of dying patients and their families by a number of social, cultural, economic, and political factors. In the 1970s, health care reformers turned to hospice as a humane alternative for the institutional care of the dying that many believed had become increasingly impersonal and technologically managed. Hospice cut across many societal boundaries and challenged assumptions about where care should be given, who should provide it, and who should be in control of the decisions surrounding that care. Yet, more than thirty years after Hospice, Inc.'s, home-care program opened, serious inadequacies remain in our contemporary model of care for the dying. Ideally, hospice interdisciplinary care teams facilitate healing in the face of separation and loss and help patients die comfortably, at home, surrounded by those who are most important to them. This is consistent with the desires of 70 percent of Americans; unfortunately, only 24.9 percent of Americans realize this wish.[114] More than one-third of dying patients spend their last days in the intensive care unit, and more than

50 percent of these patients die in moderate to severe pain.[115] The philosophical underpinnings of hospice as low-tech, high-touch integrative care for the mind, body, and spirit are gradually being supplanted by technologically driven and institutionally based medical intervention.[116]

So what can be gleaned by this historical analysis to help us understand how we arrived at this point? First, it exposes persistent societal biases that result in an overemphasis of the value of physicians and medical institutions to society, while overlooking the significance of the role that families, religious groups, and nurses have historically played in community-based care of the dying. The contemporary philosophy of hospice care evolved from a tradition of nursing care provided at home and in specialized homes for the dying. Although few of these homes were called hospices, they were critical to Saunders's conceptualization of hospice as both place and philosophy of care for the terminally ill. Saunders's medical training afforded her the requisite power and credibility to speak to physician groups and authority to lead other health professionals. Yet, it was her deep religious faith, love of nursing, and lessons she learned at St. Luke's and St. Joseph's that served as the foundation on which the hospice movement was built. As such, Saunders and other hospice advocates used a tradition of nursing care as a framework to organize, deliver, research, and reform medical care for the dying.

The study also reveals how the synergy of time, place, person, and circumstance was critical to the inception of the American hospice movement. From its inception, the movement represented the confluence of a diverse group of individuals with different motivations and interpretations of how care of the dying and bereaved should be handled. Elite hospice leaders sought to demystify the highly philosophical notions of the meaning of life and death, "being with," ministering to, and caring for dying patients and their families. Yet, it was the juxtaposition of personal ideologies, shifting professional paradigms, and social reform movements that served as catalysts to ignite and fuel the hospice movement in the United States. The civil and women's rights, death with dignity, and consumer movements laid a foundation for a growing public discourse about the quality of life, patients' rights, and the place of informed consent in the medical system.[117] Stories of how cancer patients suffered while undergoing aggressive curative treatment were widely publicized in the popular press and raised significant questions regarding the humane treatment of cancer patients. Despite the promise of curative medicine, many outside and within the health professions were beginning to wonder if the quest for cure was worth the human toll in suffering. Nursing education began to focus on alternative approaches to care, ethical and spiritual issues related to death and dying, and the hallmark of hospice, interdisciplinary teamwork.[118] The emergence of the discipline of pastoral counseling and hospital chaplains helped reintroduce faith as an important element of care for hospitalized patients. As the hospice concept was rewoven into the fabric of the American medical system, new programs developed in accordance with the personal ideologies and professional paradigms of their founders and the environment in which they were created. Although they were all committed to a similar vision of what interdisciplinary hospice care should be, each group, each discipline, and, arguably, each individual viewed what this care entailed, where it should be provided, and who should be in control through a slightly different lens.

Although Saunders served as a charismatic figurehead of the modern hospice movement, nurses and clergy were critical to its vitality in the United States. A self-identified idealist, Florence Wald provided much of the vision, passion, and courage to advance hospice as viable terminal care in the United States. Wald was in search of a way to reform care for the dying and to advance nursing within that reform. Many nurses followed her lead and became powerful forces within the grassroots hospice movement. They found strong allies in the idealistic clergy who, like Edward Dobihal, believed that the secularization of medicine had created a division among the physical, spiritual, and emotional components of care for the dying. Dobihal was searching for a way to connect the three and advance the role of clergy in the care of dying patients and their families. Although the contributions of some physicians, most notably Elisabeth Kübler-Ross, cannot be denied, for the most part the medical establishment was slow to accept the hospice concept. Whereas they endeavored to block the hospice movement in Connecticut and elsewhere, nurses and clergy led the charge for reform.

Parting Words

Throughout history, without the power base of physicians, nurses have often initiated reform on behalf of patients and families. These nurses' contributions to the improvement of the health and well-being of patients, families, and communities have been substantial. Whereas Wald's role in the advancement of hospice has recently come to light, the role of nurses in terminal-care reform predated her. The modern hospice movement was built on the legacy of nursing care provided at home and in early homes for the dying. With religion as the warp and presence as the weft, these nurses wove a rich tapestry of care for mind, body, and spirit in those early homes. Although this legacy of care has been eclipsed by the vitality of the modern hospice movement, Saunders clearly understood its comparative value when she wrote: "I do not pretend for a moment that [it] is my work. . . . Of course, most of the work is just the good nursing."[119]

Joy Buck, PhD, RN
Postdoctoral Fellow
Barbara Bates Center for the Study of the History of Nursing
and Center for Health Outcomes & Policy Research
University of Pennsylvania School of Nursing
Philadelphia, PA 19104

Acknowledgments

This work was supported by National Institute for Nursing Research: Individual National Research Service Award (F31 NR08301-01) and University of Virginia (2003–2005) and Advanced Training in Nursing Outcomes Research (T32-NR-007104) at the Center for Health Outcomes & Policy Research (2005–2007).

Notes

1. David Clark, ed., *Cicely Saunders: Founder of the Hospice Movement, Selected Letters 1959–1999* (London: Oxford University Press, 2002), 12–13.

2. Paul DuBois, *The Hospice Way of Death* (New York: Human Sciences Press, 1980); Sandol Stoddard, *The Hospice Movement: A Better Way of Caring for the Dying* (New York: Stein and Day, 1978); Lenora Finn Paradis, *The Hospice Handbook: A Guide for Managers and Planners* (Rockville, MD: Aspen Corporation, 1985); Cathy Seibold, *The Hospice Movement: Easing Death's Pains* (New York: Twayne, 1992); David Clark, "Originating a Movement: Cicely Saunders and the Development of St. Christopher's Hospice, 1957–1967," *Mortality*, 3, no. 1 (1998): 43–63.

3. Claire Humphreys, "Waiting for the Last Summons: The Establishment of the First Hospices in England 1878–1914," *Mortality*, 6, no. 2 (2001): 147.

4. Susan L. Smith and Dawn D. Nickel, "From Home to Hospital: Parallels in Birthing and Dying in Twentieth-Century Canada," *Canadian Bulletin of Medical History*, 16, no. 1 (1999): 49–64; Karen Buhler-Wilkerson, *No Place Like Home: A History of Nursing and Home Care in the United States* (Baltimore: The Johns Hopkins University Press, 2001).

5. James Walsh, *The History of Nursing* (New York: P.J. Kennedy, 1929).

6. For additional information, see Humphreys, "Waiting for the Last Summons," 146–165, Alberta Hapenny, *A Legacy of Love: A Biography of Rose Hawthorne Lathrop in Three Parts* (Pittsburgh: Dorrance 1999); Sister Mary Joseph, *Out of Many Hearts: Mother M. Alphonsa Lathrop and Her Work* (New York: Servants of Relief for Incurable Cancer,

1965); Derek Kerr, "Mother Mary Aikenhead, the Irish Sisters of Charity, and Our Lady's Hospice for the Dying," *American Journal of Hospice & Palliative Care*, 10, no. 3 (1993): 13–20.

7. See Kerr, "Mother Mary Aikenhead," and Stoddard, *The Hospice Movement*, 87. The Irish Sisters of Charity were a nineteenth-century religious order founded to care for the poor and terminally ill. Mother Mary Aikenhead, founder of the order, devoted her life to works of mercy with the poor Irish in Dublin. Roman Catholic archbishop Daniel Murray was a strong supporter of Mother Aikenhead's commitment to the "poorest of poor" and her ability to motivate others to work for the cause. In 1816, he secured papal approval for a new congregation and the Irish Sisters of Charity, an institution of women called to serve the poor and terminally ill was born.

8. Kerr, "Mother Mary Aikenhead," 14.

9. Kerr, "Mother Mary Aikenhead," 15.

10. Kerr, "Mother Mary Aikenhead," 16.

11. Humphreys, "Waiting for the Last Summons," 157.

12. Humphreys, "Waiting for the Last Summons," 159. The rules also disallowed the sisters from entering hospitals or homes of "heretics" unless there was hope of conversion to Catholicism.

13. Shirley du Boulay, *Cicely Saunders, Founder of the Modern Hospice Movement* (London: Hodder and Stoughton, 1984); Cicely Saunders, "Foreword," in Derek Doyle, Geoffrey W.C. Hanks, and Neil MacDonald, eds., *Oxford Textbook of Palliative Medicine* (London: Oxford University Press, 1993), v–viii.

14. Humphreys attributes these distinctions to middle- and upper-class morality during the Victorian Era. There were clear distinctions made between poverty and pauperism and the respectable and nonrespectable poor. It was believed that the nonworking or undeserving poor should be cared for in workhouse infirmaries. The conditions in these institutions were deliberately harsh to serve as a deterrent for reliance on them. The stigma of pauperism was used as a social tool to reduce it.

15. Humphreys, "Waiting for the Last Summons," 160–2.

16. Methodist theology and the Protestant ethic of dying was in contrast to a traditional Catholic death. Catholic deathbed rituals were intended to prepare believers for death and served as a bridge between life on earth and life in heaven. To the Methodists, dying was part of living, and as such, Protestants could achieve a good death by the art of holy living. See Shai Lavi, "The Modern Art of Dying: The History of Euthanasia in America," PhD dissertation, University of California at Berkeley, 2001.

17. du Boulay, *Cicely Saunders*, 61.

18. Humphreys, "Waiting for the Last Summons," 61.

19. For more information about the role of Catholic benevolence in health care, see Christopher J. Kauffman, *Ministry and Meaning: A Religious History of Catholic Health Care in the United States* (New York: Crossroad, 1995); and Barbra Mann Wall, *Unlikely Entrepreneurs: Catholic Sisters and the Hospital Marketplace, 1865–1925* (Columbus: The Ohio State University Press, 2005).

20. Katherine Burton, *Sorrow Built a Bridge: A Daughter of Hawthorne* (1937; New York: Image Books, 1956). See also Patricia Dunlavy Valenti, *To Myself a Stranger: A Biography of Rose Hawthorne Lathorp* (Baton Rouge: Louisiana State University Press, 1991), 131; Sister Mary Joseph, *Out of Many Hearts* (New York: The Servants of Relief for Incurable Cancer, 1981), 22.

21. Hawthorne and Huber received permission from the Dominicans to form a religious community. Rose took the religious name Sister Mary Alphonsa and Alice became Sister Mary Rose. On December 8, 1900, they professed vows as members of their new community, the Dominican Sisters, Congregation of St. Rose of Lima.

22. Hapenny, *A Legacy of Love*, 129.

23. The "quest for cure" and use of experimental treatments and surgeries in terminally ill cancer patients was of concern to Lathrop and other reformers during the early twentieth century. See, for example, Richard Cabot and Russell Dicks, *The Art of Ministering to the Sick* (New York: Ferris Printing Company, 1936). The authors discussed problems associated with care for the sick and dying in research and teaching hospitals. They listed common patient complaints about physicians and nurses, including the tendency of physicians to focus too much on research and teaching rather than on the patient.

24. Mother M. Alphonsa to Mother M. Rose, August 15, 1908, Archives of the Servants of Relief for Incurable Cancer, Hawthorne, New York.

25. Valenti, *To Myself a Stranger*, 170; Walsh, *The History of Nursing*, 270.

26. Burton, *Sorrow Built a Bridge,* 253. These words were written in a letter to James Walsh, MD, PhD, a benefactor, supporter, and historian of nursing.

27. The window remains at the entrance of St. Christopher's. Tasma's story has been repeated frequently in books and articles about Saunders and St. Christopher's. The author was told the story by Saunders in person, while looking through the window in May 2003.

28. Brompton's Cocktail was developed in 1896 when a surgeon, Herbert Snow, demonstrated that a combination of morphine and cocaine could relieve pain in cancer patients. This concoction was introduced in the early 1930s at St. Luke's, as was around-the-clock dosing. Although there was considerable interest in the mixture in the 1960s and 1970s, physician Robert Twycross asserts it has no place in modern palliative medicine, despite the almost cult-like following who believe in the mixture as a panacea for cancer pain. Although the formulations vary, Brompton's Cocktail typically contains 15 mg morphine hydrochloride and 10 mg cocaine hydrochloride per 10 ml of the cocktail. For more information about early hospice symptom-management guidelines, see Stoddard, *The Hospice Movement*, 292–305. For more information, see Ronald Melzack, Balfour Mount, and J.M. Gordon, "The Brompton Mixture Versus Morphine Solution Given Orally: Effects on Pain," *Canadian Medical Association Journal,* 120 (1979): 435–8; Cicely Saunders, "Dying of Cancer," *St. Thomas's Hospital Gazette*, 56, no. 2 (1958): 37–47; Robert Twycross, "The Brompton Cocktail," in John J. Bonica and Vittorio Ventafridda, eds., *International Symposium on Pain of Advanced Cancer, Advances in Pain Research and Therapy 2* (New York: Raven Press, 1979).

29. du Boulay, *Cicely Saunders*, 60–73.

30. Cicely Saunders, "Origins: International Perspectives Then and Now," *Hospice Journal*, 14, no. 3/4 (1999): 3. Both Clark and du Boulay detail this era of Saunders's life in some detail.

31. Cicely Saunders, "The Treatment of Intractable Pain in Terminal Cancer," *Proceedings of the Royal Society of Medicine*, 56 (1963): 95–7. There is little documentation of Saunders's research methods or statistical analysis. She often cited anecdotal evidence, patients' stories, and, beginning in 1960, pictures of patients as evidence, which raises questions about the limitations of her research.

32. Saunders, although prolific in her writing and a propagandist for palliative care, spent more time focusing on patient care, fund-raising, and administrative duties at St. Christopher's. Two of the researchers who have played prominent roles in palliative-care research are Robert Twycross and Balfour Mount. In fact, Saunders preferred the use of diamorphine instead of morphine for management of cancer pain. When the actual effectiveness was studied by Twycross, however, there was no clinically observable difference between the two drugs given orally with adjuvant treatment. See Robert Twycross, "Choice of Analgesic in Terminal Cancer Care: Morphine or Diamorphine?" Pain 3 (1977): 93–104.

33. Saunders, "The Treatment of Intractable Pain," 195. Although in Saunders's earlier writings she speaks of the compassion that the Sisters of Charity had for patients, in later descriptions she states that they were more concerned for patients' souls.

34. Saunders, "The Treatment of Intractable Pain," 195.

35. Cicely Saunders, "The Challenges of Terminal Care," in Thomas Symington and R. L. Carter, eds., *Scientific Foundations of Oncology* (London: Heinemann Medical Books, 1976), 673–9.

36. Cicely Saunders, "The Patient's Response to Treatment: A Photographic Presentation," *Proceedings of the Fourth National Symposium, Catastrophic Illness in the Seventies: Critical Issues and Complex Decisions* (New York: Cancer Care, 1971).

37. Saunders contacted various experts in cancer care, including Dr. Robert Loberfield of the New York City Cancer Committee, Professor W. Bean of the University of Iowa, and Dr. John Heller of the U.S. National Cancer Institute. See Clark, *Cicely Saunders: Selected Letters*, for more documentation of her correspondence with American scholars.

38. Cicely Saunders, "Report of Tour in the United States of America, Spring 1963," Dame Cicely Saunders Papers, Hospice History Project, Sheffield, England, box 57, folder 2/1/92, 1 (hereinafter CSHHP). Clark reports that Saunders went through a lot of trouble to develop this report and was somewhat pessimistic about how many people would want copies. She was surprised to be contacted by so many people for copies that she ran out of them.

39. Saunders, "Report," 2. There were many people she met who did not receive a copy of the report. Quite a few people requested copies of the report. In response to their queries, Saunders explained that she had sent reports to those who had given her money. It is also interesting to note that Saunders was cautioned to downplay the role of religion in hospice, although for her it was the basis of her work.

40. Other homes are in Philadelphia; Atlanta; Fall River, Massachusetts; St. Paul, Minnesota; and Parma, Ohio. To date, these homes have cared for some 92,000 patients of all creeds and races over the years – all of it free. To this day, the sisters do not accept contributions from patients or families, nor do they take government funding or insurance payments. Bills are paid from an endowment fund, investments, and public and private donations.

41. Saunders, "Report," 24.

42. Saunders, "Report," 24.

43. There were quite a few institutions in the United States, predominantly operated by religious and philanthropic groups. For example, Calvary Hospital in New York City and Youville Hospital in Cambridge, Massachusetts, were facilities dedicated solely to the care of terminally ill patients.

44. Saunders uses the word "trained" in her report. There were differences in nursing education in the United States and the UK. Saunders expressed some concern about nursing education and the move toward professionalism.

45. This finding is substantiated, at least to some degree, by a study done by Yale–New Haven Hospital by sociologist August Hollingshead and pediatrician Ray Duff, funded by the USPHS Division of Nursing. Based on observations of nurses working with patients, they noted there were discrepancies in the nursing staff's knowledge of patient diagnosis and treatment and their understanding of patients' emotional problems. See Duff and Hollingshead, "Physicians, Nurses, and Patients," in Raymond S. Duff and August B. Hollingshead, eds., *Sickness and Society* (New York: Harper and Row, 1968), 217–47.

46. Saunders, "Report," 16.

47. Saunders, "Report," 15.

48. This observation reflects the transition of nursing education from training schools to the university. It also reflects the quality of the schools she visited.

49. Hildegarde Peplau, *Interpersonal Nursing Theory* (New York: G.P. Putnam, 1952).

50. This finding reflects the influence of the psychiatric/mental health nursing movement that was flourishing at Yale at this time. Wald trained with Hildegarde Peplau at Rutgers prior to returning to Yale to creating an MS program in mental health psychiatric nursing in the late 1950s.

51. Saunders was referring to Jeanne Quint's [Benoliel] seminal research on nursing education and care of the dying, Phyllis Verhonick's research on decubitus ulcer care and problem solving, and Harriet Werley's work on the development of nursing research.

52. Saunders, "Report," 24.

53. Saunders was particularly impressed with the work of existentialist philosopher-theologians Paul Tillich and Martin Buber. For Tillich, see, for example, "Autobiographical Reflections," in Charles W. Kegley, ed., *The Theology of Paul Tillich: A Revised and Updated Classic* (New York: Pilgrim Press, 1982); "Being and Love," in Ruth Nanda Anshen, ed., *Moral Principles of Action* (New York: Harper and Brothers, 1952); Jack Mouw and Robert P. Scharlemann, "Bibliography of the Publications of Paul Tillich," in Kegley, *The Theology of Paul Tillich*, 395–423. Buber was a renowned scholar of Jewish tradition and literature. To Buber, the basis of religious faith was the relation between man and God, the relation to the eternal Thou. Within the I–Thou relationship, any statement made about God also reflected the nature of man. For example, see Martin Buber and Judith Buber-Agassi, *Martin Buber on Psychology and Psychotherapy: Essays, Letters and Dialogue* (Syracuse, NY: Syracuse University Press, 1999).

54. Florence Wald, interview with the author, tape recording, July 21, 2001, Branford, Connecticut.

55. Wald has recently won awards for lifetime achievements in hospice/palliative care from the Hospice and Palliative Nurses Association and the American Academy of Hospice and Palliative Physicians and was named a living legend by the Academy of Nursing. "Medicare Hospice Regulations" hearing before Subcommittee on Health of the Committee on Finance, U.S. Senate, 98th Congress, first sess., September 15, 1983 (Washington, DC: U.S. Government Printing Office, 1984), 12–13. Senator Durenberger, chair of the committee, gave the recognition to Wald during a committee hearing on the hospice Medicare benefit.

56. See Florence Wald, "Emerging Nursing Practice," *American Journal of Public Health*, 56, no. 8 (1966): 1252–60.

57. Wald, "Emerging Nursing Practice," 1259.

58. Wald was not the only American nurse who was concerned about the type of care afforded terminally ill patients. Starting in the 1950s, articles in the nursing literature began calling for a new approach to care of the dying and changes in nursing education. The U.S. Public Health Service Division of Nursing funded several studies on institutional care of the dying. See, for example, Jeanne Quint, *The Nurse and the Dying Patient* (New York: Macmillan, 1967); David Sudnow, *Passing On: The Social Organization of Dying* (Englewood Cliffs, NJ: Prentice-Hall, 1967); Barney G. Glaser and Anselm L. Strauss, *Awareness of Dying* (Chicago: Aldine, 1965); Barney G. Glaser and Anselm L. Strauss, *Time for Dying* (Chicago: Aldine, 1968). See also Jeanne Benoliel, "Nursing Research on Death, Dying, & Terminal Illness: Development, Present State, & Prospects," *Annual Review of Nursing Research*, 1 (1983): 101–30.

59. Wald, interview, July 21, 2001.

60. Wald, "Emerging Nursing Practice," 1259.

61. Wald, "Emerging Nursing Practice," 1259.

62. Clark, *Cicely Saunders: Selected Letters*, 87. Although some of Saunders's expenses were covered by travel grants, she was dependent on consultation fees to cover travel expenses and donations that were sent to support St. Christopher's. Issues about money appear quite often in correspondence with Wald and other Americans.

63. Both Saunders and Wald wanted the visiting professorship to be longer than six weeks, but there was not enough money in the endowment to allow for this.

64. During Saunders's stay at Yale, she met with Dr. Elisabeth Kübler-Ross and Dr. Colin Murray Parkes. These two psychiatrists would play a significant role in the advancement of terminal-care reform.

65. CSHHP, Box 57, "The Moment of Truth – Some Aspects of Care of the Dying Patient," presented at the Yale School of Nursing, April 28, 1966.

66. Wald, interview, July 21, 2001. Saunders was a prolific contributor to both medical and nursing literature during the 1960s, 1970s, and 1980s. Her philosophy was well received in nursing circles, less so in medical circles. See, for example, Cicely Saunders, "Watch with Me," *Nursing Times*, 61, no. 48 (1965): 1615–17; Cicely Saunders, "Care of the Dying," *Nursing Times*, 9 (1959): 960–1.

67. Saunders, "The Moment of Truth," 3.

68. Saunders, "The Moment of Truth," 5.

69. Publications based on research funded by the Division include Quint, *The Nurse and the Dying Patient*; David Sudnow, *Passing On: The Social Organization of Dying* (Englewood Cliffs, NJ: Prentice-Hall, 1967); Glaser and Strauss, *Awareness of Dying*; Glaser and Strauss, *Time for Dying*. See also Benoliel, "Nursing Research on Death, Dying, & Terminal Illness."

70. Duff and Hollingshead, "Physicians, Nurses, and Patients," in Duff and Hollingshead, eds., *Sickness and Society*, 217–47.

71. Letter from Florence Wald to Cicely Saunders dated October 1968, CSHHP, box 58, folder 2/1/100.

72. Interdisciplinary Study, Research Record, 10-29-1970, 1, Florence and Henry Wald Papers, Manuscripts and Archives, Yale University (hereinafter FHWYU), box 24, folder 60.

73. Interdisciplinary Study, 2–5. Many of the nurses at St. Christopher's were Anglican nuns, and the Christian religious symbols incorporated into the structure are unmistakable, even if there was not overt discussion of a particular religious paradigm. Non-Christians might well interpret this differently than Saunders.

74. Interdisciplinary Study, 3.

75. The differences in approach were immediately apparent to Dobihal, who served as director of the chaplaincy program at Yale–New Haven Hospital. Although he met with some success in changing the culture of the hospital, it was an uphill battle.

76. Edward Dobihal, "Progress Report: First Observation and Impressions of St. Christopher's Hospice" (1970), 10, Edward Dobihal Papers, Manuscripts and Archives, Yale University, box 1, folder 14 (hereinafter EDYU).

77. Dobihal, "Progress Report," 13.

78. Dobihal, "Progress Report," 15.

79. Wald, interview, July 21, 2001; Edward Dobihal, interview with the author, July 20, 2001. See also Florence Wald, "Development of an Interdisciplinary Team to Care for Dying Patients and Their Families," *ANA Clinical Conferences* (1969): 47–55; Florence Wald, "Terminal Care and Nursing Education," *American Journal of Nursing*, 67 (1979): 1762–4.

80. Steering Committee Minutes, 3/3/1971, FHWYU. Israel used social science frameworks and methods to create "meaningful communities." Her area of interest was small-group dynamics and social communication.

81. Steering Committee Minutes, 3.

82. Steering Committee Minutes, 3.

83. Steering Committee Minutes, 1–5.

84. Steering Committee Minutes, 2. In this assertion, Saunders is similar to the approach taken to spiritual care at St. Luke's Hospice. In this context, Christianity was the unifying framework rather than any specific denominational orthodoxy.

85. Steering Committee Minutes, 5.

86. Steering Committee Minutes, 4–7.

87. St. Christopher's Hospice: Discussion Group on Religious Foundation 6, September 22, 1971, EDYU, box 1, folder 3, 1–12.

88. Hospice Planning Group Steering Committee Minutes, Philosophy Statement, April 7, 1971, EDYU, box 1, folder 5.

89. Lawrence Altman, "LSD and Heroin Found Helpful in Treatment of Terminally Ill," *New York Times*, November 13, 1971, 1. LSD is one of the major drugs making up the hallucinogen class. For more information on hallucinogens, see http://www.nida.nih.gov/Infofax/lsd.html. The modern antidrug movement or "war against drugs" officially began with the Nixon administration. For more on the history of the drug wars in the United States, see David F. Musto, *American Disease: Origins of Narcotic Control* (London: Oxford University Press, 1999); for information on the counterculture during the 1960s, see Terry Anderson, *The Movement and the Sixties: Protest in American from Greensboro to Wounded Knee* (New York: Oxford University Press, 1995).

90. These concerns were well founded. There was a significant antidrug sentiment during this time, and in some areas, criminal charges were brought against physicians who ordered narcotics for patients.

91. Edward Dobihal, "Letter to Mr. C. Pierce Taylor, Executive Director, Connecticut Hospital Planning Commission" (1971), 1–3, EDYU, box 1, folder 3.

92. Wald, interview, 2001. Dobihal, interview, 2001.

93. Yo-Li Chan, "Thoughts on Facility Planning," n.d., FHWYU, 2001-M-041, box 6.

94. Yo-Li Chan, "Thoughts," 2; Hospice, Inc., "To Honor All Life: A National Demonstration Center to Protect the Rights of the Terminally Ill," appendix D, 1–2, FHWYU, Series I, box 3, folder 23.

95. Wald, interview, 2001; Dobihal, interview, 2001.

96. Hospice, Inc., "Hospice: A Vision," October 1973, 2, EDYU, box 1, folder 4.

97. Wald, interview, 2001; Dobihal, interview, 2001; Donna Diers, interview by author, tape recording, December 19, 2000, New Haven, Connecticut.

98. Florence Wald, "First Annual Hospice Staff Report," January 14, 1974, FHWYU, box 5, folder 56.

99. Joy Buck, "Rights of Passage: Reforming Care of the Dying, 1965–1986," PhD dissertation, University of Virginia, Charlottesville, 2005.

100. Wald, "Staff Report," 3.

101. Hospice, Inc., Progress Report and Program Plan Regional Hospice Development Program, January 29, 1973, 10, FHWYU, box 22, folder 11.

102. Hospice, Inc., Progress Report, 10.

103. Elisabeth Kübler-Ross, On Death and Dying (New York: Macmillan, 1969).

104. Elisabeth Kübler-Ross, On Death and Dying (New York: Macmillan, 1969).

105. Kübler-Ross, On Death and Dying.

106. Kübler-Ross's work has been criticized by some for describing the grieving process as being linear. Kübler-Ross asserts, however, that the process is neither linear nor predictable. The stages were meant to provide a framework to help professionals and lay people normalize rather than pathologize death and grief.

107. The euthanasia movement clearly had a more grassroots foundation and focused on the individual. The death-and-dying movement remained predominantly in the world of academia among philosophers, theologians, and psychologists.

108. Peter Filene, In the Arms of Others: A Cultural History of the Right-to-Die in America (Chicago: Ivan Dee, 1998).

109. Derek Gill, Quest: The Life of Elisabeth Kübler-Ross (New York: Harper and Row, 1980).

110. Hospice, Inc., Annual Report to National Institutes of Health Contract No. N01-CN-55053, September 1, 1975, 55, EDYU, box 1, folder 4.

111. For more on the development of hospice during this time frame, see Buck, "Rights of Passage," 148–223; Joy Buck, "Home Hospice Versus Home Health: Cooperation, Competition, and Co-optation," Nursing History Review, 12 (2004): 25–46.

112. "The Hospice Movement," Washington Post, February 18, 1978, A16.

113. Florence Wald, interview with author, December 18, 2000, New Haven, Connecticut.

114. Last Acts, Means to a Better End: A Report on Dying in America Today (New Jersey: Robert Wood Johnson Foundation, 2002).

115. SUPPORT Study Investigators, "A Controlled Trial to Improve Care for Seriously Ill Hospitalized Patients," Journal of the American Medical Association, 274, no. 20 (1995): 1591–9.

116. Last Acts, Means to a Better End.

117. See for example, Hugh Heclo, "The Sixties False Dawn: Awakenings, Movements, & Postmodern Decision Making," in Brian Balogh, ed., *Integrating the Sixties: The Origins, Structure, and Legitimacy of Public Policy in a Turbulent Decade* (University Park: Pennsylvania University Press, 1996); James T. Patterson, "A Great Society and the Rise of Rights-Consciousness," in *Grand Expectations: The United States, 1945–1974* (New York: Oxford University Press, 1996), 562–93; W.J. Rorabaugh, "Challenging Authority, Seeking Community, & Empowerment in the New Left, Black Power, & Feminism," in Balogh, *Integrating the Sixties*, 106–43.

118. Florence Wald, "Terminal Care and Nursing Education," *American Journal of Nursing*, 67 (1979): 1762–4.

119. Clark, *Cicely Saunders*, 12–13.

RESEARCH REPORTS

The Rise and Demise of the Colonial Nursing Service: British Nurses in the Colonies, 1896–1966

ANNE MARIE RAFFERTY
King's College London

DIANA SOLANO
King's College London

For a period of seventy years, from 1896 to 1966, the Colonial Nursing Association (CNA) (renamed the Overseas Nursing Association [ONA] in 1919) recruited 8,400 women to work as nurses throughout the British Empire. The Association operated as a recruitment agency for the Colonial Office (CO), and during its operation, recruits were sent to every dominion and territory of the Empire. Initially, the CO adopted an arm's-length approach, but during World War II it became more directly involved in overseas nurse recruitment, establishing the Colonial Nursing Service (CNS) in 1940. The CNS formalized the government's policies in relation to nurse colonial officers who were recruited through the ONA. This development ensured parity for women in the colonial service, promoting mobility across colonies and creating the conditions for international reciprocity in nurse education and training. In effect, it established a British nursing "empire," with nursing sisters leading education and training as well as implementing nursing practice in a range of clinical settings across the Empire. When the National Health Service (NHS) was established in Britain in 1948, it compounded the postwar shortage of trained nurses, creating an urgent demand for colonial nurses to staff the NHS, a trend that has continued to the present.

In this article, we trace the history of overseas nurse recruitment in Britain through the involvement of the CO and its establishment of the CNS. We explore the notion that British nurses who were recruited to work in the colonies acted

Nursing History Review 15 (2007): 147–154. A publication of the American Association for the History of Nursing. Copyright © 2007 Springer Publishing Company.

as agents of imperialism insofar as they embodied a British nursing "empire" and influenced nursing practice and professionalism internationally. We argue that the colonial history of nursing reflected wider historical colonial developments; in the rise and demise of the CNS, British overseas nursing arguably reached its zenith at the height of colonial rule and declined as colonies gained independence and fully trained indigenous nurses gradually replaced their British predecessors. It was the policy apparatus established by the CO for the unified CNS that arguably laid the foundations for the greater flow of international nurse recruitment from and to Britain, promoting greater ease of nurse migration, which would be crucial in staffing the NHS.

Nursing and Imperialism

Even a cursory excursion into the archives of bodies such as the CNA reveals the paucity of prior research into the relationship between nursing and "empire." This stands in marked contrast to the explosion of interest in the role that science and medicine played in constructing representations of imperialism. The few existing studies based on the CNA archives[1] tend to limit their scope to colonial Africa or attempt to locate the nurses within the discourse of colonial and imperial history.[2] This has, perhaps, more to do with the current interest in revisionist histories of colonial Africa under British rule than in the history of nursing per se. Insofar as nursing has been absent from colonial and imperial history until these recent revisionist studies, they are a welcome inclusion and corrective to the record. Nonetheless, there has been little attention focused on the administrative and policy links between formal government involvement and international nurse recruitment.

The fact that the CNA changed its name to the Overseas Nursing Association (ONA) in 1919 suggests that it sought to redefine itself outside the discourse of colonialism. This raises questions as to the position of nursing sisters in colonial social relations, with both the expatriate community and their indigenous patients and colleagues. The subject of imperial rule was distinctly male, so British nurses who were recruited in the early years of the CNA's operation were something of an anomaly; often, they were the only white women in the colony. For British nursing sisters, life in the colonies was often isolated and lonely; they had little support, except from the "local committee," their main point of contact with the Association, which reinforced the Victorian values of the lady nurse of good character. In sum, nurses were discriminated against in terms of their status as colonial officers, the terms and conditions of their employment, their place in the expatriate social hierarchy, and because nursing work was considered women's work. Change in overseas recruitment policy that would go some way to addressing these issues was slow to emerge.

Recruitment Criteria: Who Was the British Overseas Nurse?

A well-connected "community of friends" whose goals were entirely pragmatic established the CNA. According to the CNA's executive, the first nurses were needed to help save the lives of colonial officials and "heroes of commerce."[3] A number of recruits were attracted on account of previous missionary or family connections with the colonies. The CNA selection committee chose its first recruits on the basis of their credentials as "lady" spinsters and being women of good character, in the sense advocated by Florence Nightingale.[4] Of course, the CNA's recruitment criteria changed over time in response to a range of pressures. But, in many ways, the microcosm of the CNA reflected the wider professional arena where the identity crisis of the new nursing profession was contested during the early twentieth century. At home in Britain, the shift from "character" nurse training to professional training based on science, which emerged from the first wave of nursing reform centered on the registration debate, was hindered, in part, by conservative proponents such as those on the CNA executive committee. The CNA reinforced the vision of the new nursing public respectability because their selection of recruits was based on lady spinsters of character trained in Nightingale teaching hospitals.[5] Early records of the recruitment interviews show that they rejected qualified nurses who, in their opinion, appeared "common" but accepted those who were "rather uneducated but thoroughly respectable."[6]

Among British colonizers, the CNA nurses represented a unique minority group. They were the first women to be recruited to the colonial service, but their distinctiveness worked to divide them from other colonial officers and subject them to discrimination and domination.[7] First, because they were white women doing what was seen as "women's work," they were of low status in the colonial hierarchy and their work was undervalued. Their contracts, work conditions, and pay were all inferior to those of their male colonial official counterparts.[8] Second, the intimate and interpersonal nature of a nurse's work with expatriate and indigenous people was, paradoxically, inconsistent with the middle-class Victorian values the CNA expected of her. Even as World War I precipitated the demand for better nurse education and training, issues of class, gender, and social status still played a major part in how the CNA committee determined who was the colonial type of nurse recruit.

What is clear from the outset is that the CNA executive had only scant information about life in the colonies and, for the most part, executive members had not traveled abroad themselves. Therefore, the CNA welcomed letters from nurses as valuable sources of information about the conditions, facilities, and services provided in specific colonies. Charles Jeffries, a senior official in the CO, notes in his history of the Office that 2,189 nursing sisters were recruited to work overseas from 1922 to 1943.[9] Not all colonial nurses were sent to the tropics, but few recruits underwent training or received any form of preparation for what they might encounter in those climes. Recruitment sources appeared to favor the large teaching hospitals, despite the fact that their training courses were notoriously weak in public health, a factor much criticized during the interwar period. Although some nurses had postregistration qualifications such as health visiting, sick children's nursing, dietetics, or domestic science, these were no substitute for training in tropical diseases, which was a routine requirement for doctors. Language competence was also noted, but no demands or offers of training were made.

The CNA had three separate but interlocking strands to its work: expanding the colonial service through the work of nurses in government hospitals, providing nursing services for private institutions, and contributing to the development of so-called "native" nursing services. From 1930, colonial policy, in East Africa in particular, was recommending the spread of education as a means of promoting the economic advancement of the country: "As in the political sphere so in the social, it should be the aim to train the natives themselves to take on an ever increasing part, not only in the work of the educational, medical, administrative and other services alike, by filling in such services any posts for which individuals may increasingly become qualified, but also in the local direction of these services through the native councils already referred to."[10] Such councils were the professional registration bodies responsible for the regulation of training standards and the vehicle for reciprocal recognition of qualifications between Britain and its colonies. This approach to work overseas was promoted by the ONA, which changed its recruitment application forms in the early 1930s to include questions that attempted to probe the applicant's attitude toward working with indigenous colleagues and patients. There is a sense in which the first CNA nurses had their eyes opened to the world and other cultures, with all the complex issues that this entailed.

An ONA report to the secretary of state in 1939 saw nursing as an important cultural conduit into the local population: "through nursing the sick in native hospitals, training local nurses and welfare work among the mothers' babies, she [the European nurse] is brought closely in touch with the life of the people and her value to the colony increases as she becomes familiar with the language and customs and wins the confidence of the native people, especially of the women."[11] The separation of so-called "native hospitals" from expatriate hospital facilities meant that the nurse could potentially be a cultural conduit, but more often the evidence suggests that she was an agent of imperialism. Nurses who were well prepared in terms of language, previous experience, or family connections in the colonies often coped better and made significant contributions, improving nursing care and health education and advice where they practiced. Some nurses recorded their responses to the health problems of their patients and their attempts to adapt their practice to the conditions in the local environment, overcoming cultural barriers and a lack of appropriate resources. Some clearly demonstrated cultural sensitivity; others reveal unabashed cultural chauvinism or paternalism.

The Rise of the Colonial Nursing Service

The CO seems to have taken little active role in influencing the work of the Association until relatively late in the interwar period. Before the inception of the CNS, the ONA tended not to engage with issues such as class and race unless there was an administrative imperative for doing so. In 1932, there had been moves to streamline the business of the CO by creating a unified Colonial Service, combining the administrative and professional staffs of departments in the various colonial dependencies. A unified service was defined as one that had "a definite membership, based upon a schedule of posts normally filled by members of the Service, a standard method of entry, and a recognized system of transferability through the Colonial Empire, entrants to a Service after its institution being liable to serve in any Dependency."[12] In January 1939, the CO wrote to the ONA about its policy of the unified service, proposing to create the CNS.

When the CO formalized its involvement in overseas nurse recruitment by establishing the CNS in 1940, the nature of British nurse recruitment to overseas posts became more closely linked with the agenda of the CO and individual colonial governments. The emphasis was on exporting British nursing practice and education to indigenous populations abroad and implementing mechanisms for greater transferability of nursing sisters across the empire. Aspects of recruitment policy responsibilities were delegated to the Ministry of Labour and National Service and the Ministry of Health. The management of overseas nurse recruitment after World War II was therefore driven by supply and demand. Furthermore, the unified CNS forced the government to address issues such as recruiting black nurses to the service, transferability of appointments, and issues of equity in terms and conditions, which the ONA had largely avoided. In doing so, the unified service raised issues such as reciprocal nursing registration, education and training standards, and the professional status of nurses across the empire.

The Rushcliffe Committee on the Training of Nurses in the Colonies (1943–45) endorsed the need for a unified colonial nursing service in which a policy of recruitment from local people was to be supported by local training with the prospect of attaining a standard that would "merit reciprocal registration with the Nursing Councils in the UK."[13] These would be the vehicles through which mobility and migration could be endorsed and mediated. Subsequently, the CNA role evolved into supplying recruits for the CNS who could provide nurse training for the indigenous populations in the colonies, with the aim of creating a workforce capable of contributing to the British NHS. In 1948, the National Advisory Council on Nurses and Midwives, along with the NHS, noted: "The ultimate goal for all colonies is the development of local nurse training schools and nurses' registration to such a standard and in such a form that reciprocity with Great Britain can be obtained, and Colonial-trained nurses can take their full place as part of the British nursing profession."[14] The international reputation of the British nursing profession and concomitant number of British nurses working in the colonies reached their height during the late years of British colonial rule. In effect, the CO policy of a unified service established a de facto British nursing "empire" in the colonies, with white women nurses at the top of the nursing hierarchy. The extent to which British nursing sisters acted as agents of imperialism is open to interpretation. British nurses came to establish their international reputation, professionalism, and British nursing skills in the colonies, albeit because of the power imbalance that sought to bring Western medicine and nursing practices to the colonial territories. British nursing sisters held the leadership roles in the colonies; they were recruited not only because of their nursing experience in Britain but also to provide nursing administration in hospitals and other clinical settings and instruction, education, and training to indigenous nurses. The international reputation of British nurses had a corresponding effect on the rate of recruitment of nurses in Britain and applicants to the ONA. Applications from British nurses to work in the colonies were at their highest numbers in the late 1940s.

With the demise of the CNS in 1966, and as more colonies gained their independence, the reputation and demand for British nurses abroad was called into question as indigenous nurses took their rightful place in their own nursing services. Colonial power and hegemony assumed by British colonial officials and internalized by British nurses in the colonies were eroded over time by policy and regulatory developments in the context of postcolonial world events. But, arguably, the legacy of CO policy in establishing the CNS was that it had laid the foundations for the postcolonial international migration of nursing services.

With the demise of the CNS, there was a significant decrease in British nurse migration overseas. However, since the 1960s, there has been a steady increase in overseas nurses recruited to the United Kingdom. The British government was thus able to exploit international recruitment of nurses to staff the NHS. Furthermore, resourcing from overseas became increasingly important in the new Commonwealth.

Conclusion

British overseas nursing has its roots in imperialism and, arguably, the legacy of CNS and regulatory-body policy continues to impact international nurse recruitment today. The previous account attempts to locate the current dilemmas associated with the international recruitment of nurses to the United Kingdom within a wider historical context. A key consideration is the ethical dilemma of exacerbating "brain drain" in skill-depleted countries, and a distinction needs to be drawn between aggressive actions by governments to recruit and individuals' decisions to migrate.[15] The current exodus of nursing staff from many poorer ex-colonies is putting increased pressure on critically depleted health care systems. Yet, it is not just governments that need to consider the policy implications of international recruitment. Nurses and their organizations need to acknowledge the degree to which they may have colluded with and benefited from overseas recruitment in the expansion of their own professional "empire." It seems that the legacy of the first migration of British nurses, who went overseas to fulfill their own dreams and play their part in the imperial mission, cautions us to take what lessons we may draw from the continuities and ruptures in the historical evidence.

ANNE MARIE RAFFERTY, DPhil, MPhil, BSc, RN
Head, Florence Nightingale School of Nursing & Midwifery
King's College London
James Clerk Maxwell Building
57 Waterloo Road
London SE1 8WA

DIANA SOLANO, PhD, MSt, BA, RN
Research Fellow, Florence Nightingale School of Nursing & Midwifery
King's College London
James Clerk Maxwell Building
57 Waterloo Road
London SE1 8WA

Notes

1. Dea Birkett, "The 'White Woman's Burden' in the 'White Man's Grave': The Introduction of British Nurses in Colonial West Africa," in Napur Chaudhuri and Margaret Strobel, eds. *Western Women and Imperialism: Complicity and Resistance* (Bloomington: Indiana University Press, 1992), 177–88; also Helen Callaway, *Gender, Culture, and Empire: European Women in Colonial Nigeria* (Urbana: University of Illinois Press, 1987), 83–109; Pat Holden, "Colonial Sisters: Nurses in Uganda," in Pat Holden and Jenny Littlewood, eds., *Anthropology and Nursing* (London: Routledge, 1991), 67–83.

2. Margaret Jones, "Heroines of Lonely Outposts or Tools of the Empire? British Nurses in Britain's Model Colony: Ceylon, 1878–1948," *Nursing Inquiry,* 11, no. 3 (2004): 148–60; Helen Sweet, "'Wanted: 16 Nurses of the Better Educated Type': Provision of Nurses to South Africa in the Late Nineteenth and Early Twentieth Centuries," *Nursing Inquiry,* 11, no. 3 (2004): 176–84.

3. "Colonial Nursing Association," *The Times,* December 2, 1898, 2.

4. Anne Marie Rafferty, *The Politics of Nursing Knowledge* (London: Routledge, 1996), 27, 38–41, 54–5.

5. Rafferty, *Politics of Nursing Knowledge,* 40–1, 68–95.

6. CNA Archives, Rhodes House, University of Oxford, Mss. Brit. Emp. s400 (hereafter CNA Archives), Register of Nurses, Bound Volume 100, for example, register numbers 195 and 241.

7. Anne Marie Rafferty, "International Recruitment of Nurses and the Colonial Nursing Service: The History of the Present," in Margaret Pelling and Scott Mandelbrote, eds., *The History of Medicine from Early Modern England* (London: England Ashgate, in press).

8. Colonial Office Paper, Establishment of a Colonial Nursing Service 1936, Public Record Office, London, CO 850/84/12.

9. C. Jeffries, *Partners for Progress: The Men and Women of the Colonial Service* (London: G. Harrap, 1949), 152.

10. Memo on Native Policy in East Africa, 1930, cited by Janet Welch in "Nursing Education Related to the Cultural Background in East and Southeast African Colonies," CNA Archives, box 141, item 1.

11. Observations of the Committee of the Overseas Nursing Association Regarding the Colonial Nursing Service, February 9, 1939, CNA Archives, box 133, file 4, 14–17.

12. Observations of the Committee, February 9, 1939, 7–8.

13. Colonial Office, Committee on the Training of Nurses for the Colonies: Minutes and Papers 1943–1945, Public Record Office, London, CO 998/30/11.

14. National Advisory Council on Nurses and Midwives, "Training of Colonial Student Nurses in the United Kingdom," Scottish Records Office, Edinburgh, HH103.348 Paragraph 9(iii), 1948.

15. James Buchan, Tina Parkin, and Julie Sochalski, *International Nurse Mobility: Trends and Policy Implications* (Geneva: World Health Organization, 2003).

RESEARCH AND COMMENTARY

Florence Nightingale's Opposition to State Registration of Nurses

CAROL HELMSTADTER
University of Toronto

It is well known that Florence Nightingale strongly opposed state registration for nurses. Her opposition is usually treated in the standard literature as reactionary and dismissed in a few paragraphs. For example, Dock and Stewart wrote in 1931 that, when state registration was first publicly broached in 1887, Nightingale had reached the point "where the old cannot go on with the young," adding that "no doubt her years of seclusion made it difficult for her to realize the newer conditions."[1] Nightingale was actually sixty-seven years old in 1887. In this article, I argue that although Nightingale did adhere to an older ideal of nursing as a religious vocation, a view that was becoming less acceptable to young women in the 1890s, she was a lady of extraordinary perspicacity and had many reasons for opposing state registration that were realistic, well informed, and intelligent.

First and foremost, Nightingale understood that nurses in the late 1880s and 1890s were simply not educated well enough to be registered as a profession. Second, the proponents of state registration wanted to exclude working-class nurses and make nursing a profession for ladies only. Nightingale believed many of the most competent nurses were working-class women. Third, she believed the campaign leaders did not distinguish adequately between medicine and nursing and were placing nursing under the control of medical men. Fourth, she found the state registration proposal for credentialing inadequate. Finally, she was distressed by the dishonesty and lack of professional ethic on the part of the campaign's leaders. Throughout the whole debate, Nightingale's focus would be on clinical competence and expertise, while the state registration party would focus on improving the social status of nurses.

Nursing History Review 15 (2007): 155–166. A publication of the American Association for the History of Nursing. Copyright © 2007 Springer Publishing Company.

The Campaign for State Registration

The British Nurses Association

Ethel Bedford Fenwick, former matron of St. Bartholomew's Hospital, led the lobby that was pushing for state registration. Bedford Fenwick was a flamboyant, ambitious, and competent person who had been a great success as matron and would later become the primary founder of the International Council of Nurses. Full of spirit and with a will of steel, she was rich, well educated, and beautiful,[2] but Dr. Norman Moore, who taught the course on medical nursing at St. Bartholomew's, believed her to be unscrupulous and wanting in honor. One of the City of London companies had given the hospital a prize to be awarded to the probationer who achieved the highest score on her final exams. By the late 1880s, these companies, descendants of the medieval guilds, were largely charitable organizations that supported community activities. Bedford Fenwick waited until she had seen the marks the doctors gave each nurse, and then added marks for good conduct to those of her favorite nurse so as to give her the top score. The case was so flagrant, Moore said, that the doctors asked the company for another equal prize. Nightingale was not certain that Bedford Fenwick's addition of points for conduct was wrong. "Perhaps a matron would be right," she commented. A St. Bartholomew's nurse had told her that if any nurse did something wrong, Bedford Fenwick was sure to know about it before the next morning. "All satisfactory evidence is that Mrs. Fenwick was unscrupulous but generally right," Nightingale concluded.[3]

In 1887, Bedford Fenwick and a group of matrons, including Catherine J. Wood, former matron of the Hospital for Sick Children in Great Ormond Street, founded the British Nurses Association (BNA), the organization that would lobby for state registration.[4] Wood would become Bedford Fenwick's second-in-command in the early years of the campaign. Wood, Mr. William Scovell Savory, one of the consulting surgeons at St. Bartholomew's, and Dr. Bedford Fenwick, Ethel's husband, began furiously canvassing Nightingale to join. Wood also told Lucille Pringle, matron of St. Thomas's, that she was "bound in honor" to become a member. Pringle sent a letter declining to do so, but at a large BNA meeting, with Princess Christian, one of Queen Victoria's daughters, in the chair and Pringle herself in the audience, the BNA read out Pringle's name in the list of members. "They are absolutely unscrupulous," Nightingale exclaimed.[5]

In October 1888, the BNA General Council claimed 1,146 members, with requests from New Zealand and New South Wales to form chapters.[6]

A year later, it published a list of several thousand members. This figure can be compared with the approximately 50,000 nurses listed in the 1891 census. The 1889 BNA list was full of inaccuracies: a number of the nurses on the list had never been trained at the hospital where they claimed to have been trained, a number had started training at the hospital they named but had not finished, and a large proportion had simply been employed at the hospital but not enrolled in its training school. Others had been discharged for inefficiency or misconduct.[7]

The Goals of the British Nursing Association

In April 1888, the BNA began publishing its official journal, the *Nursing Record*. The articles in this journal demonstrate the BNA's naive concept of state registration and one of its major goals: eliminating working-class nurses. BNA leaders believed that state registration would elevate nurses "instantly into a *profession* recognized by the law" and that nurses would then rank immediately with other professions authorized by the state.[8] In their view, registered nurses would automatically acquire better social standing and better pay, while the legislation would outlaw nurses who practiced with inadequate training. Such nurses would be open to criminal prosecution and probably given a term of hard labor.[9] More gentlewomen would then enter the profession, relieving the nursing shortage. Within ten years, nursing students, like medical students, would have to pay for their training.[10] (Tuition fees, of course, would have made nurses' training unaffordable for working-class women.) Nursing thus would become an occupation exclusively for ladies because the state registration party believed only those who had "a liberal education, largely gained by contact with educated men and women, and a refined home training" were really able to acquire the powers of observation and sympathy that were essential to a good trained nurse.[11]

The BNA leaders planned to use the Medical Act of 1858 as the model for their proposed registration act.[12] The 1858 act established a register of medical men with a General Council that was self-governing and that could dismiss members of the profession for failure to perform up to standard. To gain admittance to the register, a doctor had to pass the requirements and examinations of one of twenty-one already established licensing bodies.

The legislation the BNA was seeking indicates how poorly its leaders understood the 1858 Medical Act. The act did *not* establish new licensing bodies, it did *not* outlaw unregistered practitioners, and it did *not* try to remove practitioners on the basis of their class or social graces. Although what the Victorians called

quacks and other unqualified practitioners were perfectly free to continue practicing, the act did restrict some of their activities such as prescribing potentially
dangerous drugs.[13] "The BNA knows neither the legal, professional, social or
financial difficulties" of bringing in such legislation, Nightingale wrote in 1889.
Such an act, she said, would make nursing a legal profession but a profession
without legal rights.[14]

Nightingale's Arguments

Written Examinations

Nightingale's best-known argument against the BNA plan for state registration
was its dependence on a written examination the nurse would have to pass to
gain admission to the register. In fact, Nightingale did not object to written examinations as such. Her first concern was that such exams tested only memory.
They could not test what for Nightingale were the more important factors: the
nurse's personal and moral character and her nursing practice. Written exams
could not test a nurse's ability to apply her knowledge on the ward, her appreciation of the different character of each individual case, or the individuality of each
patient.[15]

   Nightingale had always been doubtful of the validity of written examinations
as a test of performance. When discussing army reform forty years earlier – in the
late 1850s – she opted against the use of competitive exams. The civil service had
been reformed in the early 1850s, using competitive exams for both recruitment
and promotion, and the government was considering applying this system to
the army. In Nightingale's view, public opinion in the army itself judged fairly
correctly the merits of its officers. "If I, with my superficial knowledge of the
Crimean Army, could give you a tolerably correct idea of the fitness of general and
commanding officers there for command, is it credible that the Commander-
in-Chief could not arrive at a just judgment generally?" she asked. "The qualities that you really want," she continued, "viz. self-control, self-reliance, habits
of accurate thought, integrity and what you generally call trustworthiness
are not decided by competitive examination, which tests little else than the
memory."[16]

   Second, Nightingale was very aware of the major barrier written examinations posed to working-class nurses. Until 1870, most working-class children
had only a smattering of schooling, usually two or three years of grade school.

Forster's Education Act of 1870 had made primary education much more available, and in 1880, elementary education was made compulsory, although it was not until 1891 that it became completely free.[17] Because probationer nurses usually had to be twenty-three when they entered training, the cohort that benefited from the 1880 and 1891 acts—that is, those who had completed elementary school—would only begin working their way into the training schools in the 1890s. Nightingale thought that nurses as a body were simply not well enough educated to undertake state registration.[18] Registration, she said, would only be appropriate for nurses in the future.[19] "You cannot register what is not there," she wrote. The wide variation in the competencies of nurses presented another problem. If the good were registered together with the indifferent, the indifferent would obviously predominate; so, Nightingale said, registration that was supposed to raise the standard would instead lower it.[20]

Nursing for Ladies Only

In 1888, Nightingale put out a pamphlet, "Is a General Register for Nurses Desirable?" She published it under the name of Henry Bonham-Carter, her cousin, and the Secretary of the Nightingale Fund Council because she believed it would be divisive to publicly identify herself with one party or the other. She argued that upper-class women had an unfair advantage on written exams because they were better educated and therefore more accustomed to expressing their knowledge in words. They would do far better on written exams than less well-educated but clever nurses whose nursing knowledge might be as good and whose fitness for the work possibly better. The upper-class nurses would get better positions as a result of their higher scores, whereas the less educated nurses would get second-rate positions. This would be an injustice to working-class nurses and a great loss to the nursing profession.[21]

The *Nursing Record*, in response, was enraged. The author was ignorant of the facts, it editorialized; he thinks it does not matter whether a nurse drops her *h*s; whether she is pretty or plain, her caps and aprons charming or ugly; or whether she was bred in the drawing room or the scullery. "What an estimate of nursing qualities and position," the lead editorial declaimed.[22]

The BNA was well aware of the three severe structural problems in the nursing workforce about which Nightingale wrote: the very poor level of education of most working-class women when they entered training; the tiny amount, or absence, of education in most so-called training schools; and the difficulty recruiting nurses. The BNA's solution to these problems, as we have seen, was simply to get rid of the working-class nurses to make the occupation so much more attractive to ladies that they would flood into the profession, solving the nursing shortage. In the same way, if the ladies paid for their nursing education, their tuition fees would provide better funding for the training schools, enabling them to improve the instruction.

Nightingale was more realistic about these difficulties. There were already ladies, known as lady or paying probationers, who did pay fees for their training, but they were few and far between. Even in the two most fashionable training schools, St. Bartholomew's and St. Thomas's, usually only one-fourth to one-third of the probationers were ladies.[23] At all the hospitals except St. Thomas's, in fact, many paying probationers came for only three to six months and then left.[24] If there were no working-class nurses, there would be practically no nursing workforce. The shortage of nurses was of long standing, antedating the early nursing reforms. From at least the beginning of the century, there had been great difficulty attracting able women into the occupation, and now, Nightingale pointed out, in the 1890s, other spheres of work for educated women were opening and attracting many of the first-rate women who had formerly gone into nursing,[25] a factor that could only aggravate the supply problem.

The Line Between Nursing and Medicine

Nightingale objected strenuously to the way the BNA failed to differentiate nursing from medicine and the way it placed nurses and their training schools under the control of doctors. State registration, Princess Christian explained at the opening meeting of the BNA, would make nursing "a legal profession inseparable from the profession of medicine."[26] Similarly, the *Nursing Record* stated that nursing would be a distinct profession and "an inseparable part of the noble profession of medicine,"[27] somewhat of an oxymoron. D.P. Griffon in her discussion of Bedford Fenwick and state registration argues that Bedford Fenwick's two main convictions were first, that only trained women should be allowed to call themselves nurses, and second, that hospital administrators and antagonistic doctors should not be allowed to exploit nurses. Doctors should not credential nurses; nurses should be the gatekeepers of nursing. At the same time, Griffon says, Bedford Fenwick appreciated that the membership of learned medical men would enhance the standing of the BNA.[28]

But the membership of the learned medical men enabled them to influence the credentialing of nurses. To secure the backing of these men, the BNA

General Council agreed unanimously to adopt a circumscribed, or what they called practical, educational program. This was to reassure the doctors that theoretical knowledge would not predominate in nurses' training and possibly threaten medical supremacy. What was this practical education that was to be the uniform curriculum for the registered nurse? The only abstract part of the lengthy curriculum was "some knowledge of elementary anatomy and physiology." The rest all dealt with practical activities: sweeping, dusting, polishing, changing sheets, dressings, leeches, blisters, sick cookery, taking temperatures, and the various ways of disinfecting clothes, rooms, and utensils.[29]

Doctors had a powerful voice in the BNA. The General Council of the Association consisted of Bedford Fenwick as permanent president, her husband, Dr. Bedford Fenwick, as treasurer, other nurse founders as vice presidents, a hundred medical men, a hundred matrons, and a hundred sisters or nurses. By April 1888, the BNA was boasting that it had a predominance of doctors as members – 500 doctors and 90 matrons, a claim that seems somewhat unlikely. Its executive committee, which it would later expand and make somewhat more representative, consisted of Princess Christian, eleven doctors, and twenty-two matrons or equivalents, while doctors usually chaired the BNA meetings.[30] Organizing nurses under the control of their natural leaders – medical men – is the very essence and *raison d'être* of the BNA, an editorial of the *Nursing Record* declared in 1889.[31] It is a well-known fact, a later editorial explained, that "the BNA was founded chiefly, if not entirely, by the assistance of the medical men; that from that time until now it has been mainly dependent on their exertions."[32]

These doctors made the position of nurses vis à vis medicine very clear. Nurses should be "absolutely docile, skilful and submissive, unbiased by habit and without self esteem," Dr. Octavius Sturges, physician to the Westminster Hospital and a member of the BNA, explained in a lecture at a BNA meeting in 1889. They should demonstrate the deference to the doctor that the female gender owes to the male. Doctors ordered and nurses executed. Nurses should demonstrate wisdom rather than knowledge and use simple speech, not the doctor's scientific vocabulary.[33] Yet, where nursing education was concerned, Sturges was one of the more advanced doctors. Although he believed some doctors gave too much scientific detail in their nursing lectures, he also believed nurses should be allowed to listen to the discussions senior doctors had with their medical students as they made their rounds in the wards.[34] Traditionally, this had been forbidden.

Nightingale was not at all happy with the BNA positioning of nursing. Nurses should not be placed under medical men, she said.[35] It was extremely dangerous to put the new training schools under the control of the BNA, where doctors had such a strong voice.[36] Doctors did not know what a good nurse is, Nightingale scoffed, and besides they were terrible administrators.

Credentialing

Although the BNA was prepared to grandfather lady nurses such as Bedford Fenwick and Wood, who had had only a year or less of training, it ruled that after January 1, 1889, all nurses admitted to the register must have three years of training.[37] Nightingale objected to this proposal for two reasons. First, she said, no hospital could afford to give three years of real training to its probationers. Those hospitals that claimed to do so usually offered instruction only in the first year and used the probationer as a full-time staff nurse in the last two years.[38] Among the many costs of training nurses, suitable accommodation was perhaps the most expensive. At St. Thomas's, with its Nightingale Fund money, there was a comfortable Nurses' Home, but even there, adequate space to house more than one class of probationers, much less three, was not to be found.[39] Second, in terms of nursing education, the BNA was as aware of the uneven quality of the hospital training schools as Nightingale. When the BNA decided to make a three-year hospital certificate the criterion for admission to their register, she pointed out the inconsistency of their position. "Who is to certify the hospitals?" she asked.[40]

The proposed BNA Registration Board included many doctors and retired matrons like Bedford Fenwick and Wood, whereas Nightingale believed only experts – people currently working and training the nurses and who knew them personally – should credential nurses. They should be certified individually rather than by a standardized examination.[41] Although the BNA sought the trappings of a profession, Nightingale concentrated on professional practice and proposed what was essentially an apprenticeship model, the model so looked down on by later nursing leaders.

Yet, as Tom Olson and Eileen Walsh indicate in *Handling the Sick*, there is a strong apprenticeship legacy in nursing that deserves historical legitimacy.[42] And, of course, apprenticeship was an important part of almost all the new nineteenth-century professions such as architecture, engineering, and accountancy. The learned professions of law and medicine also retained strong apprenticeship features. Nightingale's preferred model was more like that of medicine. By the late 1880s, medical education had moved into the academy, but each professor had his house surgeon or physician and medical students whom he supervised and instructed on the wards. Medical students wrote exams, but they were also examined individually by senior doctors in a clinical setting.[43]

Conclusion

"It [state registration] is a formidable movement which I regret," Nightingale wrote in 1888. "It will do the nurses great harm."[44] Indeed, when state registration was finally introduced in 1919, her prediction that it would make nursing a professional body but a body without legal rights[45] proved entirely correct. The close alliance with a group of doctors who were determined that nurses be entirely dependent on medical orders for every act would prove strangling to the nascent profession.

Joan Lynaugh points out that the proregistration party failed to examine their assumption that state registration was the best route to professional recognition.[46] In contrast, Nightingale examined that supposition closely and was convinced that nursing could only become a profession through professional education. An Act of Parliament introducing a register for nurses could not professionalize nursing, she said. Rather, first the nurses had to professionalize themselves by becoming better educated.[47] Margarete Sandelowski highlights the way nurses today are frequently obliged to carry out some core practices illegally.[48] We are still battling for control of our own practice, Ellen Baer points out.[49] Nurses do not have what Patricia D'Antonio calls the cultural authority to match their critical clinical responsibilities.[50] This began in the nineteenth century. Nightingale's judgment that if registration came too early it would do great harm to the profession proved prescient.

CAROL HELMSTADTER, RN (RET), BScN, MA
Adjunct Assistant Professor
Faculty of Nursing
University of Toronto
34 Chestnut Park
Toronto, ON M4W 1W6
Canada

Notes

1. See Lavinia L. Dock and Isabel M. Stewart, *A Short History of Nursing from the Earliest Times to the Present Day* (New York: G.P. Putnam, 1931), 130–1.
2. Susan McGann, "Ethel Gordon Fenwick 1857–1947," *Oxford Dictionary of National Biography* (http://www.oxforddnb.com/); Susan McGann, *The Battle of the Nurses: A Study of Eight Women Who Influenced the Development of Professional Nursing, 1880–1930*

(London: Scutari Press, 1982), 54; Winifred Hector, *The Work of Mrs. Bedford Fenwick and the Rise of Professional Nursing* (London: Royal College of Nursing, 1973), 35–6.

3. Florence Nightingale (hereafter FN), Notes on visit of Dr. Norman Moore, February 24, 1888, British Library Additional Manuscripts (hereafter BL Add. MSS) 47761, ff 30–9.

4. Brian Abel-Smith, *A History of the Nursing Profession* (London: Heinemann, 1960), 68–9; FN, Notes on meeting with Lucille Pringle, July 12, 1889, BL Add. MSS 47722, ff 16–17.

5. FN, Notes on meeting with Pringle, ff 15–20.

6. *Nursing Record,* October 18, 1888, 398.

7. FN, Notes for Mr. Rathbone, 1889, Hampshire Record Office, 94M72(f582/43).

8. Editorial, *Nursing Record,* June 14, 1888, 121–2 (emphasis original).

9. *Nursing Record,* June 14, 1888, I: 121–2; W.J. Mollett, "Legal Status of Nurses," *Nursing Record,* April 5, 1888, I: 5–7.

10. Editorial, *Nursing Record,* May 24, 1888, 86–7.

11. Miss Mollett, "Culture," *Nursing Record,* June 14, 1888, 125–7; C.M. Loch, "What Constitutes an Efficient Nurse?" *Nursing Record,* May 10, 1888, 64–7.

12. *Nursing Record,* April 5, 1888, 2.

13. W.J. Reader, *Professional Men: The Rise of the Professional Classes in Nineteenth Century England* (London: Weidenfeld & Nicolson, 1966), 63–8.

14. FN, Notes on visit with Sir James Paget, July 13, 1889, BL Add. MSS 47755, ff 71–4.

15. FN to Louisa Mary Elizabeth, Grand Duchess of Baden, April 6–16, 1896, BL Add. MSS 47750, ff 184–5.

16. FN to Lord Stanley, May 17, 1857, Liverpool Record Office, 920 Der 15/1.

17. R.K. Webb, *Modern England from the Eighteenth Century to the Present* (London: Unwin Hyman, 1980), 344–5.

18. FN, Notes, February 21, 1888, BL Add. MSS 47755, ff 41–6.

19. FN, Notes on meeting with Paget, ff 71–2.

20. FN to Henry Bonham-Carter, May 22, 1891, BL Add. MSS 47723, ff 173–7.

21. Henry Bonham-Carter, "Is a General Register for Nurses Desirable?," reprinted in toto in *Nursing Record,* September 6, 1888, 301–4.

22. Editorial, *Nursing Record,* August 9, 1888, 233–5.

23. List of probationers, September 18, 1889, BL Add. MSS 47739, f 101; List of Probationers, June 1894, BL Add MSS 47741, f 147; Register of Nurses 1879–1905, Archives of St. Bartholomew's Hospital, SBH/MO52.

24. Evidence of Sir Sidney H. Waterlow, *Parliamentary Papers,* 1890, XVI: 164–5; Abel-Smith, *Nursing Profession,* 31–2.

25. FN to Louisa Mary Elizabeth, Grand Duchess of Baden, April 6–16, 1896, BL Add. MSS 47750, ff 184–5.

26. *Nursing Record,* April 5, 1888, 2.

27. *Nursing Record,* April 19, 1888, 26.

28. D.P. Griffon, "Crowning the Edifice: Ethel Fenwick and State Registration," *NHR,* 3 (1995): 203–4, 206.

29. Report on Meeting of the General Council of the BNA, *Nursing Record,* October 18, 1888, 398–402.

30. *Nursing Record,* April 5, 1888, 2, 5–9; see also October 18, 1888, 398.

31. Editorial, *Nursing Record,* July 11, 1889, 18.

32. Editorial, *Nursing Record,* March 6, 1890, 109–10.

33. Dr. Octavius Sturges, "Nurses and Doctors," Part I, *Nursing Record,* March 28, 1889, 197–9.

34. Sturges, "Nurses and Doctors," Part II, *Nursing Record,* April 4, 1889, 213–15.

35. FN, Notes, June 19, 1893, Clendening Library, University of Kansas.

36. FN to Henry Bonham-Carter, April 28, 1891, BL Add. MSS 47723, ff 152–5.

37. Abel-Smith, *Nursing Profession,* 69–70.

38. *Parliamentary Papers,* 1892: lxxxiv–v.

39. FN to Sir Henry Acland, July 22, 1893, London Metropolitan Archives H1/ST/NC1/93/6; FN to Henry Bonham-Carter, August 8, 1892, Hampshire Record Office, 94M72/f 582/22.

40. FN, Notes, February 21, 1888, BL Add. MSS 47755, ff 41–6.

41. FN, Notes for Rathbone, Hampshire Record Office, 94M72/f582/43.

42. Tom Olson and Eileen Walsh, *Handling the Sick: The Women of St. Luke's and the Nature of Nursing, 1892–1937* (Columbus: The Ohio State University Press, 2004), 153–5.

43. J. R. Ellis, "The Growth of Science and the Reform of the Curriculum," in F.N.L. Poynter, ed. *The Evolution of Medical Education in Britain* (London: Pitman Medical, 1966), 155–68; W.R. Merrington, *University College Hospital and Its Medical School: A History* (London: Heinemann, 1976), 76–9.

44. FN to Maude and Fred Verney, February 16, 1888, BL Add. MSS 68885, ff 175–6.

45. FN, Notes on meeting with Paget, ff 71–2.

46. Joan Lynaugh, "Common Working Ground," in Barbara Mortimer, ed., *New Directions in Nursing History: International Perspectives* (London: Routledge, 2005), 195.

47. FN, Letter to Eva Lückes, April 7, 1889, London Hospital Archives PP/Luc/1.

48. Margarete Sandelowski, "The Physician's Eyes: American Nursing and the Diagnostic Revolution in Nursing," in Ellen D. Baer, Patricia D'Antonio, Sylvia Rinker, and Joan E. Lynaugh, eds., *Enduring Issues in American Nursing* (New York: Springer, 2001), 224.

49. Ellen D. Baer, "Contemporary Issues in Historical Context," in Baer et al., eds., *Enduring Issues,* 3–9.

50. Patricia D'Antonio, "The Nature or Power and Authority in Nursing," in Baer et al., eds., *Enduring Issues,* 147–9.

Commentary

Linda Holbrook Freeman
University of Louisville

Florence Nightingale has been a symbol of the caring, high moral character, and culture of gentlewomen that came to characterize the image, if not the reality, of modern nursing. But, later critics have dismissed both her personal attributes and her contributions, concluding that her vision for nursing, rather than enhancing, actually delayed and misdirected the development of the profession. The subordinate position of nursing in relation to physicians, the failure to educate nurses in universities, and the delay of implementing a system for licensing and registration of nurses are given by her critics as examples of her negative influence on both the nursing profession's early development and current status. Her legacy has been debated by scholars, and at times this debate has spilled over into the public arena, particularly in Britain.[1]

Carol Helmstadter's article examines one of those examples critics have cited: Nightingale's opposition to the state registration of nurses. Although Nightingale's own complicated calculus of economic, legal, professional, educational, political, and social issues led to her stated opposition to the campaign, she also, as Helmstadter points out, believed that the timing was not right.

Helmstadter also argues that another reason underlying Nightingale's opposition was the character and aims of the lobby for registration. Although examples are cited that describe unprincipled behaviors on the part of Ethel Bedford Fenwick, a leader in the campaign for registration, the conclusion that these behaviors form Nightingale's argument against registration are not fully supported. Clearly, Nightingale was not a supporter of Fenwick or the movement, nor did she personally value the behaviors cited. However, the author notes that Nightingale was able to conclude that Fenwick, even if unscrupulous, was generally right in one instance described. There is clearer support for other reasons for Nightingale's opposing the British Nurses Association plan for state registration than the issue of Fenwick's character.

It is the impact of Fenwick's leadership, evident in her work in the British Nurses Association and in the *Nursing Record*, which she edited, that is a pervasive thread in Helmstadter's narrative. In her analysis, Fenwick's leadership clearly underscores Nightingale's opposition, which was, in part, a reaction to Fenwick's proposals. But, Nightingale was able to move beyond her personal mistrust of

Nursing History Review 15 (2007): 167–168. A publication of the American Association for the History of Nursing. Copyright © 2007 Springer Publishing Company.

Fenwick's character to concentrate on the underlying issues of nurse registration as proposed. We might look instead at Nightingale's place in the social context of the campaign to more fully understand her opposition.

The author's comprehensive approach to understanding the debate over registration between these two nurse leaders provides an excellent summary, both of Fenwick's campaign and of Nightingale's opposition. What is lacking in this approach is an analysis of the social context that drove the campaign. The entry of women into the workforce, increasing feminist thought, and philanthropy played critical roles in the social context that provided the momentum for the kinds of change that registration of nurses represented. Nightingale's view of nursing as a religious vocation, only briefly mentioned in the article, was an important factor in her opposition to nurse registration. This view of nursing reflected her mystical experiences and the influence of the Evangelical movement of the nineteenth century and deserves exploration. This movement compelled both men and women to do good work. The importance of philanthropy was critical in the development of social work, including nursing, as a legitimate role for women. This, in conjunction with the demands for an increased labor force that included the need for women workers and the feminists' focus on resolving women's exclusion from employment opportunities, helps explain both the proposal for and the opposition to nurse registration. Further consideration of workforce issues, the women's movement, and Nightingale's view of nursing as a calling by God would help broaden and clarify her stance on opposition to state registration of nurses.

LINDA HOLBROOK FREEMAN, RN, DNS
Professor
School of Nursing
University of Louisville
Louisville, KY 40292

Note

1. See, for example, Christopher J. Gill and Gillian C. Gill, "Nightingale in Scutari: Her Legacy Reexamined," *Center for International Health,* 40 (2005): 1799–805. In addition, *The Times* of London carried a story on the vote of a British labor union to "ditch Florence Nightingale as the patron saint of nurses." "*Nurses Ditch Florence Nightingale as Patron,*" *The Times,* April 27, 1999: 11. This story was followed by multiple letters to the editor, published in *The Times,* May 3, 1999: 21. Later, *The Times* ran a brief note questioning whether Florence Nightingale was a heroine, "*Hero. . .* " *The Times,* November 16, 2004, Public Agenda 7. See also "The BBC *vs.* Florence Nightingale" (*Reputations: Florence Nightingale, Iron Maiden,* BBC2, July 17, 2001) for a review of controversy over a film broadcast by BBC.

BOOK REVIEWS

Nightingales: The Extraordinary Upbringing and Curious Life of Miss Florence Nightingale

By Gillian Gill
(New York: Ballantine Books, 2004) (535 pages; $27.95 cloth)

How did the young, well-bred, Florence Nightingale become the Florence Nightingale memorialized as heroine, founder of modern nursing, and statistician? Most who know of Nightingale's work focus on her post-Crimea life. But Gillian Gill, who has also authored biographies of Agatha Christie and Mary Baker Eddy, decided to explore Nightingale's life *before* she chose to enter the public arena. What results is a rich, readable, and entertaining narrative that analyzes Nightingale and her family within the military, political, and social contexts of eighteenth- and early-nineteenth-century England.

Gill's central thesis is that one cannot understand Nightingale's choices, strengths, or flaws without considering her family background and childhood. Drawing on numerous primary sources concerning Nightingale and her extended family and friends, Gill suggests that most biographers have uncritically accepted Nightingale's version of her early life, particularly the lack of family support for her interest in nursing. Gill convincingly argues that Nightingale's family, although often exasperated by her choices, continued to love her, missed her when she traveled, and put up with a lot from her. In many Nightingale biographies, Florence's mother, Fanny, and sister, Parthenope, exist as negative mirrors to Florence's nontraditional choices and ambitions. Gill, however, draws a much deeper portrait, and as a result, we see certain events through their eyes, not just from young Florence's perspective. The detailed examination of Nightingale's family history, childhood, and the way in which her father structured her education also help us understand why she was drawn to nursing rather than to medicine.

The book begins by tracing her father's and mother's families back through the eighteenth century. Nightingale's progenitors included both male and female reformers who participated in reform movements relevant to their era, for example, by joining slavery abolition groups and participating in the religious radicalism of the English Protestant Dissenters. We learn of her parents' courtship and travels, Nightingale's privileged Victorian childhood, and her emerging young womanhood in the context of Victorian society's constricted opportunities for women. Gill also examines closely the first defining act of Nightingale's life, her rejection of marriage to a man about whom it appears she cared deeply, Richard Monckton Milnes.

It is not until the second half of the book that Nightingale seeks training at Kaiserworth and employment at Harley Street. Ultimately, she embarks for Crimea, where many aspects of the oft-told story are interwoven with new details, such as Nightingale's relationships

Nursing History Review 15 (2007): 169–209. A publication of the American Association for the History of Nursing. Copyright © 2007 Springer Publishing Company.

with other women present in the war zone. Gill's book ends where many other Nightingale biographies begin warming up: when she returns from the war zone and becomes an invalid. There is an epilogue, however, that summarizes the ensuing decades in which Nightingale did much of her work.

The author manages to present a portrait of Nightingale that depicts her many flaws and inconsistencies without detracting from her accomplishments or debunking her legitimacy as a heroine. One distinct strength of this work is that Gill provides ample analysis of the way in which gender, class, and other variables shaped Nightingale's actions. She is able to do so without immersing her arguments or conclusions in academic jargon or cumbersome prose that might make the book less accessible or interesting to the general reader.

This book should enthrall anyone with a curious mind who enjoys a good read. For those who want to understand women's place in Victorian England, a consideration of this book would be useful. But the work also has something specific to say to nurses of all ages, backgrounds, and specialties. Most of us enter nursing, like Nightingale, wanting to do something meaningful with our lives. By considering how Nightingale, wittingly and unwittingly, drew from the successes and failures of earlier generations of her family's women, we are encouraged to consider our own past and the ways in which it has shaped our particular present. Because Nightingale emerges as a "real" woman in the drama, one with flaws, neuroses, and contradictions along with many strengths, instead of a sanctified, sanitized one, any nurse who hopes to make a difference in the world is reassured that perfection is not a prerequisite to caring; and shrewdness, ambition, and political savvy are not impediments.

CYNTHIA CONNOLLY, PhD, PNP
Assistant Professor
Yale University School of Nursing
Assistant Professor, History of Medicine and Science
Yale University
100 Church Street South
P.O. Box 9740
New Haven, CT 06536

Bermerkungen zur Krankenpflege (German translation of *Notes on Nursing*)

By Florence Nightingale, with commentary by Christoph Schweikardt and Susanne Schulze-Jaschok
(Frankfurt am Main: Mabuse-Verlag, 2005) (276 pages; 24,80 Euro)

Bermerkungen zur Krankenpflege is a new German translation of Florence Nightingale's *Notes on Nursing*, which was published in 1860. There were two German translations within a year of the first English publication and a third translation in 1868. Christoph Schweikardt and Susanne Schulze-Jaschok believe that Nightingale's vision in *Notes on Nursing* is relevant for our time and have attempted to produce another translation that is accessible to a wider audience and, at the same time, more faithful to Nightingale's spirit and style than earlier translations.

To give *Notes on Nursing* greater cogency for a twenty-first-century reader, the authors provide a preface of five short essays. These essays begin with a three-page overview of Nightingale's life and work, focusing on her life leading up to *Notes on Nursing*. Her whole life is presented in table form toward the end of the book (pp. 256–258). The second essay describes the social characteristics and living conditions of the working class in mid-nineteenth-century England. Public health reforms are presented in light of the state of scientific knowledge at that time. This places Nightingale's work as a sanitarian within its historical context and her relationship with Edwin Chadwick and William Farr, who were leaders in the public health movement. In the third essay, the authors discuss Nightingale's ideas about health and disease and how her religious beliefs were integral to these ideas. They demonstrate that her ideas, although out of step with modern germ theory, were not out of step with mid-nineteenth-century science. The authors also contrast the understanding of contagion and infection as presented in the *Notes* with our modern conception. The fourth essay on the meaning and lessons of caregiving is basically a synopsis of the *Notes*. The fifth essay is a short discussion of Nightingale's view of the ideal nurse and her belief that nursing was a "calling," not simply an occupation. Nightingale stated her difficulty in describing the good nurse as other than "devoted and obedient" (p. 18), a definition that will raise the hackles of a modern nurse. These essays create a mind-set for reading *Notes on Nursing* with a depth of understanding. The preface ends with a list of five books for further reading, four in English and one in German.

This very readable text meets the authors' goal of maintaining the flavor of Nightingale's own writing, and it is accessible to a wide audience. A medical glossary (pp. 259–265) and a table of equivalences in weights, measures, and money (p. 266) assist in understanding the text today.

The epilogue examines the status of research on Nightingale and places this new translation within the context of recent scholarship. Nightingale remains a fruitful field for research and writing; and, since the 1980s, there has been a shift from the earlier hagiographic view of her. The authors use the works of Monica Baly[1] and Hugh Small[2] as examples. They take issue, however, with Small's claim that *Notes on Nursing* was in reality "directed *against* doctors, hospitals and nursing care." They were unable to discover support for this interpretation anywhere in Nightingale's work (p. 239). The book ends with a bibliography and a list of Internet resources.

Translating a nineteenth-century English text into a twenty-first-century German one is at the same time converting to another cultural context and a different time frame. One is also moving from a Christian-based culture to a secular culture. Citing Scott Montgomery,[3] the authors believe that a "translation is always at the same time an interpretation," "eine Übersetzung immer gleichzeitig eine Interpretation dar" (p. 244). They reject the earlier translations (Victor Skretkowicz's[4] analysis of Nightingale's three English versions of *Notes on Nursing* and the nineteenth-century German translations) that were based on word for word and phrase for phrase, which they refer to as "imitation of syntax structure," "die Nachahmung syntaktischer Strukturen" (p. 246). Instead, they opt for comprehension and readability for the German reader. At the same time, they show how they have remained true to the way Nightingale appealed directly to her readers. This analysis of previous translations and the description of their own method is the most interesting section of the book.

The translation of *Notes on Nursing* is a pleasure to read and, coupled with the preface, makes reading the *Notes* meaningful to an educated general public and to undergraduate students. The epilogue will be helpful for graduate students and scholars. The use of so many English references suggests a paucity of material written in German, making this text especially valuable to a German audience. Schweikardt and Schulze-Jaschok have created a comprehensive resource and a significant edition to the Nightingale literature.

Joyce Schroeder MacQueen, BN, MEd, MSc.
Associate Professor (Retired)
Laurentian University
5627 Clearwater Lake Road
Sudbury ON P3G 1L9
Canada

1. Monica Baly, *Florence Nightingale and the Nursing Legacy* (London: Croom Helm, 1986).
2. Hugh Small, *Avenging Angel* (London: Constable, 1998).
3. Scott L. Montgomery, *Science in Translation: Movements of Knowledge Through Culture and Time* (Chicago: University of Chicago Press, 2000).
4. Victor Skretkowicz, *Florence Nightingale's Notes on Nursing* (London: Baillière Tindall, 1996).

Turn Backward, O Time: The Civil War Diary of Amanda Shelton

By Kathleen S. Hanson

(Roseville, MN: Edinborough Press, 2006) (160 pages; $14.95 paper)

Amanda Shelton is one of the many courageous and exceptional women usually grouped among "background" figures mentioned in the accounts of women who provided nursing care in the Civil War. Kathleen S. Hanson's book, *Turn Backward, O Time*, presents Shelton's personal diary, which chronicles her experiences as a Civil War diet nurse for the Christian Commission and other work from 1864 to 1866.

As a twenty-one-year-old woman, Shelton, along with thousands of other women, volunteered her services, motivated in part by patriotic zeal and religious principles, to ease the sufferings of the sick and wounded Union Army soldiers. Shelton left her home in Iowa to become a "diet nurse," a new concept for the treatment of ill and wounded soldiers. Stationed primarily in the Tennessee area, she oversaw the preparation of the special foods required by the physicians for the hospitalized soldiers. Her diary chronicles the day-to-day activities of the diet kitchen, her struggles with the physicians who viewed this work as unnecessary and saw the diet kitchen and nurses as a threat to their authority, and her observations of the surrounding area and the people she met in differing circumstances. Juxtaposed in her writings are her impressions of the sights and smells of war: "The wounds smelled so bad that I almost vomited" (p. 74). Shelton followed in the same date entry with a description of the surrounding area: "Three of us walked up to the top of Lookout today.

Birds hopped among the branches and sang as gleefully as though there were neither sin nor war in this beautiful wicked world" (pp. 74–75). Throughout her diary, she intersperses her private thoughts with reflections on God, using Bible phrases and hymn verses to bring a sense of understanding and acceptance to the scenes she witnessed.

Shelton's diet nurse experiences lasted only eighteen months, when she was removed by her mentor, Anne Wittenmeyer, from her hospital in Nashville for attending dances at the hospital where she worked – considered unseemly behavior in a nurse, compounded by her attendance in the company of a married man, the physician in charge of the hospital. Only alluded to in Shelton's entry, further explanation of these incidents is contained in letters at the end of the book by the physician involved and by Wittenmeyer. However innocent the activity of dancing in a hospital where there were wounded soldiers, the precarious position of women in a war zone necessitated the removal of Shelton to safeguard the efforts of the other women who were nursing the soldiers.

The book concludes with an address given by Shelton on her experiences as a Civil War nurse to a reunion of Spanish-American War veterans and nurses in 1908 and before another group in 1911. She acknowledged the "superior training" of the Spanish-American War nurses but stated, too, that she and her Civil War contemporaries "hath done what she could."

Hanson provides a thorough and comprehensive introduction of Shelton's life that presents an explanatory background to her diary, which brings clarification to the diary entries that would otherwise appear as unconnected and unexplained thoughts. Without this introduction, the diary would be an unremarkable contemporary record of a young woman's nursing experience instead of the richer description of the perspective of wartime nursing and the woman who gave this care.

Turn Backward, O Time represents another excellent addition to the growing bank of historical documentation about individual women and their unique nursing contributions in the Civil War, which laid the foundation for the development of modern nursing and nursing education in the United States. Amanda Shelton's diary provides an up-close glimpse of an extraordinary young woman, volunteering to serve with the noblest of intentions in the bloody conflict of the Civil War, and maturing and coming of age in the harshest of environments for a woman of her era. Her thoughts and writings provide a window of discovery into a woman who, despite witnessing the horror of the aftermath of battle, still found hope and promise in caring for others. This book represents an invaluable contribution to those desirous of studying Civil War nursing, nursing in wartime, women's history, and one woman's personal thoughts and recollections of all she witnessed.

TERESA M. O'NEILL, RNC, PHD
Associate Professor of Nursing
Our Lady of Holy Cross College
New Orleans, LA 70131

Unlikely Entrepreneurs: Catholic Sisters and the Hospital Marketplace, 1865–1925

By Barbra Mann Wall

(Columbus: The Ohio State University Press, 2005) (344 pages; $49.95 cloth)

Unlikely Entrepreneurs, Barbra Mann Wall's long anticipated history of Catholic nursing sisters, has been well worth the wait. This ambitious and successful work breaks new ground by positioning Catholic sisters as absolutely central to the larger histories of institutions, clinical practice, health care policy, immigration, and women's care work. In addition, *Unlikely Entrepreneurs* definitively shifts our historiographical focus from urban East Coast hospitals to the much more paradigmatic health care institutions established by Catholic sisters throughout the American heartland. In sum, we now know that the nursing women we have too often taken for granted built and operated (and, in many instances, still do operate) much of the American hospital system. We have a more gendered story of hospital formation, a more nuanced method of analyzing the interplay between the secular and the philanthropic missions of health care institutions, and a deeper appreciation of the importance of ethnic ambition in structuring caregiving roles and in creating community institutions.

Unlikely Entrepreneurs focuses on the work of three orders of Catholic nuns: the Sisters of St. Joseph of Carondelet from St. Paul, Minnesota; the Sisters of Charity of the Incarnate Word from San Antonio, Texas; and the Sisters of the Holy Cross from Notre Dame, Indiana. Between 1865 and 1925, these three orders alone operated and/or owned more than forty hospitals in the Midwest and the Trans-Mississippi West. In Wall's telling, these orders were deeply engaged in a capitalistic medical marketplace with an entrepreneurial ethos that allowed them to establish, market, finance, and administer increasingly complex hospital networks *and* advance Catholic spirituality and values. There were few dichotomies or contradictions in the sisters' sense of entrepreneurship. Rather, commercialized exchange and religion were deeply integrated: the more financially stable the hospital, the greater the social and spiritual returns. But, the end purpose of the nuns' entrepreneurship, Wall argues, was fundamentally different than that of other market institutions: the goal for the nuns was not to expand profit and market share but to protect and advance Catholicism where it might be threatened. Success was measured in lives saved, deaths eased, and baptisms.

Part 1 lays out the background of these religious entrepreneurs. Many, if not most, had family roots in the working-class Irish immigrant experience, and they saw themselves as missionaries in a country dominated by Protestantism. These women also belonged to orders directly responsible to the pope rather than the local bishop: local communities (or dioceses) could request the nuns' help, but they could not order it. These women took vows that committed them to anonymity, but this was an anonymity deeply embedded in a powerful collective identity that emphasized the specialness of their place, that created a certain élan about suffering and sacrifice, and that elevated hard and servile work to a holy apostolate. These women were celibate, and their celibacy, in Wall's mind, was their most important departure from traditional gender roles: by deliberately de-emphasizing gender – in their dress and in their taking of male saint's names – they created a space where they could work that was devoid of sexual connotations.

Part 2 brings us deeper into the hospitals that these Catholic sisters created. The capitalistic medical marketplace, as Wall argues in a comparison of successful and unsuccessful hospital ventures, was a risky and perilous place. Her sisters had to compete: with other hospitals caring for patients from other social groups; for patients who could pay for their care; for physicians who would treat patients; and for the limited amount of government monies that might subsidize the care of poor patients. Market conditions and community support were critical: in Utah, for example, St. Joseph's Hospital closed when the mines shut down, while Holy Cross thrived along with the adjacent Salt Lake City mines and railroads. But, the sisters' ingenuity and business acumen (and tight control over escalating costs) also played critical roles. They pioneered prepayment plans that would cover workers' hospital costs. In direct opposition to the more traditional system of appointing attending physicians, they kept their medical staff appointments open to all community physicians who would continue to treat (and charge) their now-hospitalized patients. They also aggressively marketed an image of their hospitals as an interrelated (rather than dichotomous) sacred *and* scientific place containing the best technology, ruled by sexual discipline, and untarnished by mercenary self-interest.

Wall also considers the sisters' hospitals as social places when she compares them to the non-Catholic hospitals in similar regions. She suggests that the sisters' hospitals were, like others, very much of a particular time and place. Her sisters never engaged in any public discussion about the causes of poverty. And, although slightly more progressive in their practices, they never challenged the prevailing attitudes about race. They segregated black and Mexican patients, for example, but in many places only the sisters' hospitals would admit African Americans, and their Mexican patients were often treated by physicians from their own community.

Part 3 moves us to a more systematic analysis of the interplay of religion, gender, and autonomy in the sisters' hospitals. Religion was at the heart of the sisters' nursing care, and nursing the sick and dying created sacramental situations that linked the worldly and the divine. As Wall points out, a drink of holy water could be at once a source of miraculous intervention, spiritual restoration, and relief. The sister-nurses brought a particularly American Catholic ethos that recognized the inevitability of pain and suffering to the routine day-to-day aspects of care that replicated that of most other hospitals. A sense of a "good death" – one that centered on the Church's sacraments and the return of a lapsed soul back into the fold – was important to the nuns. It could often, though, be a source of criticism of their care. Wall quotes Thomas Dwight, a physician and Catholic convert, who asserted in 1895 that the sisters' hospitals "may have been the best place for a Catholic to die in; they were not the best for him to get well in" (p. 145).

But, the centering of authority in the hands of religious women was the most unique and unprecedented aspect of the sisters' hospitals. The sister-administrators appointed physicians, negotiated contracts, controlled admissions and discharges, and reserved the right to make the final decisions about all matters related to the hospital. Most often, sister-administrators preferred negotiation and compromise in the face of conflict: they understood their need for public association with the social prestige of physicians. Also, the sister-administrators were well aware of Church and social prescriptions: they often used the language of obedience, humility, and self-effacement to fashion a more acceptable presentation. But, when necessary, these women could and would balance the increasing power of medicine with their own spiritual power. In Wall's words, "as 'brides' of Christ and representatives of the Catholic Church, nuns had their own special status, and no layman could rival it" (p. 151).

But, as the twentieth century advanced, the sisters found themselves and their hospitals under increasing pressure to professionalize, modernize, and, to some extent, secularize. The increasingly influential standards set by the American College of Surgeons gave physicians more authority and control over the hospitals; the new Catholic Hospital Association recognized the sisters' accomplishments but denied them appointments as officers; and new requirements for professional nursing education and practice all posed unprecedented challenges. The sisters' adapted, but the most dynamic years of profound autonomy and influence were drawing to a close. As Wall wonders in closing this important work, in the modern hospitals' de-emphasis of the spiritual component of health care and healing, have we lost more than we gained?

PATRICIA D'ANTONIO, RN, PHD, FAAN
Adjunct Associate Professor of Nursing
Barbara Bates Center for the Study of the History of Nursing
University of Pennsylvania
Philadelphia, PA 19104

When Matron Ruled

By Peter Ardern
(London: Robert Hale, 2002) (256 pages; $32.50 cloth)

"Nurses, in the last resort, were not expected to exercise independent judgment and were, in fact, expressly restrained from doing so, which was one reason why so many people thought it such a suitable profession for women,"[1] wrote W.J. Reader in his 1966 study of the professions in England in the nineteenth century. In short, with the inability to exercise professional judgment, Reader did not think nursing could be considered a real nineteenth-century profession. Peter Ardern's study, *When Matron Ruled,* places the Victorian model of nursing superintendent squarely within this context. His work describes an important part of the nursing ethos and demonstrates the way so many of the nurses who worked under these authoritarian matrons admired and respected them. "It must all seem rather harsh now," one of the nurses Ardern interviewed explained, "but nurses knew where they were, and who their leader was, and liked it" (p. 244). Twentieth-century Victorian-style and authoritarian matrons, whom Ardern calls the "last dinosaurs," disappeared from the British hospital scene shortly after Reader made his comments.

Although it includes a bibliography, this is not a historian's work in that it does not have the scholarly apparatus of footnotes. This is to be regretted because the author has consulted many archival collections and conducted extensive interviews of retired matrons and their families. The oral histories are the strength of the book, making it required reading for those who want to understand an important part of nursing's cultural heritage. The interviews make the chapters on twentieth-century nursing the most useful. Especially valuable are the descriptions of the Cinderella services. The stories of workhouse masters and matrons are particularly interesting. In some workhouses, these positions were still exclusively reserved for married couples well into the twentieth century. The chapters on military nursing, notably those on the Falkland and Gulf wars, are a major contribution to the literature. There is also a wonderful collection of pictures, which are a delight to anyone interested in nursing history. The photograph on the dust jacket of a matron lining up her nurses with a ruler is wonderful in the way it illustrates the concerns and character of the old-style matron.

The author, a psychiatric nurse with a PhD in health studies who later worked as a counselor to the elderly, sets out to defend the leadership style of the old-style matron and to indicate the wide range of her roles. Ardern sees the frequent stereotype of the matron as a battle-axe or a dragon as a misrepresentation and believes she was really a fine nursing professional "who could impose order on doctors, nurses, patients and relatives, such was the awe and esteem she was held in" (p. 204).

Despite Ardern's effort to reverse the dragon image, he writes admiringly of her as "a terrifying sight," whose constituency regarded her with fear and awe as she swept into the ward "like a battleship." Her strict, authoritarian discipline ensured safety, efficiency, and high standards at all levels – asepsis, infection control, bedside care—while moral authority was maintained by "those dreaded visits to matron's office" (pp. 164–165). The causes of the visits that are mentioned here seem to have little to do with patient care but rather were for failure to have one's cap perfectly pleated or because it was worn somewhat askew, or for breaking a thermometer. The portrayal of matron as *in locis parentis* comes across as somewhat hypocritical, for she turned a blind eye to the student nurses who were breaking the strict dormitory rules, and indeed, in a chapter on "The Other Side of Matron," she is described as sometimes leading a double life herself, a life that would not have gibed with the rules she was supposed to be imposing on her nurses. Ardern explains this inconsistency by saying that these strict regulations were necessary because young women until the 1960s and 1970s were immature and unworldly wise.

One wishes that Ardern had engaged with Brian Abel-Smith's penetrating question in his classic 1960 *History of the Nursing Profession*: did the petty restrictions and regulations and the harsh discipline encourage good patient care? How often, Abel-Smith wonders, did the junior nurses, operating beneath "the sceptre of fear" and themselves victims of authoritarianism, unconsciously treat their patients in the same way? Nor does Arden address Abel-Smith's point that while other young women in the twentieth century were leaving behind Victorian restrictions, the Victorian discipline that the "last dinosaurs" imposed was a major cause of the persistent shortage of nurses. It would also have been interesting to see Ardern deal with Martha Vicinus's construction of the Victorian matron in her chapter on nursing in *Independent Women*. A debate on these issues could enhance the defense of the old-style matron.

Historians will wish that the author had asked the classic historiographical question of "why" more often. This is particularly relevant to the disappearance of the old-style matrons. Ardern details what was lost when this position was removed from the hospital structure – a culture of dedication, allegiance, leadership of a certain kind, a superintendent who had started at the bottom and risen through the ranks, and the loss of camaraderie as university education replaced the old hospital training schools. Certainly, all of these factors had real value and were indeed lost, but why were these matrons phased out if they were such highly respected and essential persons? "Matrons showed great adaptability and enthusiasm for change. Matron had been flexible to meet new demands and challenges, but without compromising standards in nursing. Matrons were the much-respected and feared giants of hospitals, the stalwart leaders of nursing," Ardern explains. "Like many other things in our careless modern world, matrons were unable to survive the climate of change, a change to a new organizational and management structure of nursing" (p. 238). If matrons truly were giants, flexible and adaptable, enthusiastically welcoming change and essential to the hospital organization, why were they unable to maintain their positions? The author does not deal with contextual issues that made this type of matron appropriate in the nineteenth century but inappropriate in the twentieth century, when not only organizational and management structures, which he mentions, had changed, but also the social and economic position of women was making this particular Victorian style of leadership obsolete.

As depicted in *When Matron Ruled*, one could not disagree with Reader's conclusion that nurses cannot be considered professional in the modern sense of the word. Under the rule of the old matrons, nurses offered a service to the public certainly, but their leaders, as presented here, seemed more interested in appearance and strict discipline than in supporting or developing a specialized body of knowledge that would provide nurses with the professional judgment to act independently. This is not to say that many nurses did not develop highly sophisticated professional judgment, but this portrayal of the old matrons suggests that they did not support or encourage this thrust. We must be grateful to Ardern for documenting this aspect of nursing history and for capturing so well the atmosphere in the world of the old matrons.

CAROL HELMSTADTER, RN (RET), BScN, MA
Adjunct Assistant Professor
Faculty of Nursing
University of Toronto
34 Chestnut Park
Toronto, ON M4W 1W6 Canada

1. W. J. Reader, *Professional Men: The Rise of the Professional Classes in Nineteenth Century England* (London: Weidenfeld & Nicolson, 1966), p. 181.

Latter-day Saint Nurses at War: A Story of Caring and Sacrifice

By Patricia Rushton, Lynn Clark-Callister, and Maile K. Wilson
(Provo, UT: Religious Studies Center, Brigham Young University, 2005)
(296 pages; $29.95 cloth)

Wartime nursing is a true test of the strength of the human condition. The writings of Elizabeth Norman's *We Band of Angels: The Untold Story of American Nurses Trapped on Bataan by the Japanese*[1] and Evelyn Monahan and Rosemary Neidel-Greenlee's *And If I*

Perish: Frontline U.S. Army Nurses in World War II [2] are tributes to the profession of nursing and vividly describe the experiences of nurses who do the work of nursing during wartime. Similarly, in *Latter-day Saint Nurses at War*, authors Patricia Rushton, Lynne Clark-Callister, and Maile Wilson state that the purpose of their book is to "tell the story of Latter-day Saint nurses who have served during wartime situations" (p. 1). In so doing, this contributory history adds to the scholarship of both women's and nursing history.

Published by the Religious Studies Center at Brigham Young University, *Latter-day Saint Nurses at War* is written for a lay audience. It begins with an introduction that highlights notable figures in biblical times who have cared for others in times of need. Nursing leaders such as Florence Nightingale and Clara Barton, who helped establish nursing as a profession, are also highlighted in the next chapters of the book as the authors set the stage for Mormon women who practiced nursing. In this section, the authors also emphasize the importance of collecting and archiving the stories of Latter-day Saint nurses who have practiced during wartime, fearing that their histories would otherwise be lost. Unlike Norman, Monahan, and Neidel-Greenlee, who focused on nurses' practice during one war, Rushton, Clark-Callister, and Wilson feature selected nurses who share a common faith across eight decades of international conflict. It is an ambitious project, and as such, lacks intimate details to truly capture the featured nurses' experiences.

The authors divide their work into chapters chronologically by wartime conflict, beginning with World War I and ending with Operation Iraqi Freedom. In each chapter, nurses' experiences during these conflicts are described through anecdotal excerpts from their diaries or letters home to their families. In many of the cases, the authors conducted interviews with the nurses themselves to capture the memories of their wartime work. In each section, a summary of the events surrounding the circumstances leading to war precedes the cameo of the nurses' experiences in order to place the featured nurses within an historical context.

In their discussion of the historical background of each chapter, the authors rely on secondary-source citations. In many instances, there is no segue between the historical background and the profiles of the nurses who practiced during that time in history, which makes the work somewhat choppy. Still, the quotations and stories of the featured nurses are always moving and inspiring no matter what the era. For example, Nurse JoAnn Coursey Abegglen is featured in the Vietnam War chapter. Nurse Abegglen gives a detailed account of her childhood and describes a selection of her memories of wartime nursing while in the Air Force Reserves. She stated, "We never let anybody die on our flights," and she mentioned burned patients on the plane (p. 171). There is no information, however, on how she helped stave off death or how she treated the burn victims. Indeed, the wartime experience of each nurse could easily evolve into a book of far greater detail.

It is difficult to write contemporary history because we lack the necessary time and space that offers perspective on these events. To their credit, however, the authors capture and record the experiences of nurses not only in past wars but also of those who cared for casualties of the recent tragic events and conflicts associated with the attacks of September 11, 2001, and the current Iraqi War. These narratives can be useful for future archival research.

The strength of the book lies in its survey of lesser-known nurses who are often not included in general histories. Although they portray the wartime experiences of almost seventy nurses, across more than eighty years, the authors are modest in their use of referenced material and fail to truly make connections either between the nurse and the war or the nurses themselves. This work would have been strengthened by the inclusion of the location of the archival material, a discussion of how the nurses were identified, and more detailed descriptions of their actual practice during war. As it stands, the narratives and archival material speak for themselves, and it is up to the reader to analyze them and enjoy this celebration of the practice of nursing.

The book highlights how the nurses' Mormon faith assisted them in overcoming the harshness of wartime conditions and the devastating losses faced by those around them. What is needed next is an analysis of how Mormon women's nursing experiences relate to broader issues concerning the role of religion and culture in American society.

JENNIFER M. CASAVANT, RN, MSN, ACNP-BC
Doctoral Candidate
University of Virginia School of Nursing
Charlottesville, VA 22911

1. Elizabeth M. Norman, *We Band of Angels: The Untold Story of American Nurses Trapped on Bataan by the Japanese* (New York: Pocket Books, 1999).
2. Evelyn Monahan and Rosemary Neidel-Greenlee, *And If I Perish: Frontline U.S. Army Nurses in World War II* (New York: Alfred Knopf, 2003).

Alcoholism in America: From Reconstruction to Prohibition

By Sarah W. Tracy

(Baltimore: The Johns Hopkins University Press, 2005) (xxiii + 357 pages; $48.00 cloth)

Sarah W. Tracy begins her history of the changing medical and cultural definitions of habitual drunkenness with the founding of the American Association for the Cure of Inebriates in 1870 and concludes with the implementation of the Eighteenth Amendment in 1920. Throughout, she explores the changing ways in which physicians, psychologists, the general public, and inebriates (author's term) themselves characterized the problem as both a medical diagnosis and a moral issue. Tracy does not mention nurses or nursing care; instead, she is interested in the diagnosis of alcoholism and its social and cultural framework. She explores a variety of sources, including medical and institutional records, legislative debates, minutes of temperance groups, published articles, and advertisements. Through such records, she concludes that diagnosis and treatment were not top-down processes of medical imperialism but rather negotiations among physicians, patients, and the public. She clearly demonstrates that defining and treating habitual drunkenness involved medicine, as well as understandings of gender, class, ethnicity, and social order.

Tracy locates the changing terminology used to describe habitual drunkenness and the proprietary and state-sponsored treatment options in the context of medical, social, and cultural history. She argues that several factors during the Gilded Age and Progressive Era combined to make the question of inebriety one of widespread concern at that particular time. For example, industrialization made workplace efficiency and safety pressing concerns; urbanization and immigration brought large numbers of people to cities with various ideas about alcohol; and state welfare reform efforts and the professionalization of medicine led to the creation of asylums. Even while a scientific, medical conception took hold, however, chronic drunkenness continued to hold moral connotations of personal failure, weakness, or sin.

During the period discussed, four terms reflected developments in the medicalization of chronic drunkenness. The first, *intemperance*, implied individual volition and held the most moral connotations and ties to the temperance movement. *Dipsomania* came into use around the turn of the twentieth century and connoted the most innocent view of the "habitual drunkard." The term denoted a hereditary disease similar to insanity that afflicted the more sensitive nervous systems of the middle and upper classes. The most common term, *inebriety*, encompassed many forms and types of addiction, including periodic and chronic addictions to alcohol or other substances. This was a psychiatric condition that encompassed the mind, body, and morals. *Alcoholism* first took hold in the early twentieth century, partly as a more specific form of *inebriety*. The term shifted the focus from person to substance, although it did not remove all connotations of blame from the person.

Inebriety was also characterized as a disease of modern civilization, one caused by a fast pace of life, urbanization, poverty, immigration, and changing gender roles. Sobriety, then, was not only a means of healing the inebriate but also a means of restoring the social and domestic order. Recovery for men meant restoring their masculinity, something attained through a "fight" to recover. Even more so than males, however, female inebriates threatened the social order by violating social understandings of respectable womanhood. These women were synonymous with loose morals, sexual promiscuity, and ruined motherhood. Indeed, they were viewed as a threat to the nation's future generations.

Treatment options also reflected the increasing medicalization of inebriety. Individuals could find "cures" in stores or through the mail, although most physicians did not believe that such treatments were effective. Instead, they advocated city and state facilities designed specifically to treat inebriates rather than sending them through the penal system or to mental hospitals. Although Tracy acknowledges that homes for inebriates, private asylums, cures, and public inebriate hospitals varied in their approaches to treatment, she argues that they all treated inebriety holistically as a medico-moral disease. She details the specific methods of each option and spends two chapters comparing the state treatment facilities of Massachusetts and Iowa. This is an interesting comparison that highlights the importance of local culture. In Massachusetts, for example, the contexts of industrialization, urbanization, and immigration figured more importantly than in Iowa, where restoring the patient to become a productive member of the agricultural society was a more important goal. Tracy concludes with an exploration of inebriates' views of their disease as a medico-moral one. By exploring patient correspondence and published narratives, she finds that they often saw the telling of their story as part of their own treatment, as well as a means of helping others.

Tracy's book is well argued and supported, although at times needlessly repetitive. It clearly adds to the historiography of medicine, yet it is relevant for historians of many fields, including nursing. Her connections between the history of inebriety and its social contexts illustrate how historians of all fields can benefit through the study of social and cultural history. For nurses in particular, her work demonstrates that to fully comprehend any disease, nurses need to know how attitudes about the disease are constructed and how they change over time. Other studies could certainly follow in this model, for, as Tracy argues, "disease is not just clinical pathology; it is social commentary" (xi).

Kara Dixon Vuic, PhD
Assistant Professor of History
Bridgewater College
Bridgewater, VA 22812

Unnatural Selections: Eugenics in American Modernism and the Harlem Renaissance

By Daylanne K. English
(Chapel Hill: University of North Carolina Press, 2004) ($49.95 cloth)

In *Unnatural Selections*, Daylanne K. English, a professor of African-American literature, argues that eugenics, the science of breeding better humans, was a pervasive component of early twentieth-century American culture. It permeated the social sciences, medicine, and politics. Eugenics affected public policy, popular culture, and American literature. The early twentieth century has variously been termed the "Progressive Era" by historians, "modernism" by American literary scholars, and the "Harlem Renaissance" by African-American historians and literary scholars. In this interdisciplinary, cross-racial cultural study, English asserts that the content of the various writings in this period in American history was shaped by new national struggles such as immigration, migration, and intraracial breeding.

English examines the similarities and differences of eugenic ideology and its challengers as seen in literary, medical, and sociological texts. Furthermore, through the works of vastly disparate writers such as W.E.B. DuBois, T.S. Eliot, Gertrude Stein, "New Negro" female playwrights such as Angelica Weld Grimke, and white female eugenics field workers, English argues that modern American literature mirrored the social, political, and scientific climate of the day. She justifies her selection of DuBois, Eliot, and Stein as being representative of the American modernist movement, the Progressive Era, and the Harlem Renaissance according to contemporary literary scholars. Along the lines of Gail Bederman's *Manliness and Civilization*,[1] English emphasizes the "shared intellectual contexts of white and black modern writers" (p. 22), while recognizing that these writers' own personal conditions (race, gender, and social class) influenced their thinking and writing.

In the introduction, English traces eugenic thinking and its utopian roots back to England's nineteenth-century social philosopher Herbert Spencer and social scientist Sir Francis Galton. She explains how this ideology spread to America and made its way into all facets of American life. Then, in the first three chapters, specific writers and their texts are analyzed. In Chapter 1, the writings of the influential African-American leader W.E.B. DuBois are examined. Editor of the NAACP's magazine entitled *Crisis*, DuBois championed African-American uplift and fought for civil rights long before the term was coined. At the same time, English argues, DuBois was a proponent of eugenic thinking, as evidenced by his racial uplift discourse. In a 1922 edition of *Crisis*, for example, DuBois states: "...In time efficiency and brains and beauty are going to be well-bred in the American Negro race" (p. 48). This was not racist, according to English. However, it *was* elitist: DuBois envisioned a "better social and political future" (p. 64) for people of color that could be achieved through aesthetics and selective reproduction. In Chapter 2, English examines the modernist author T.S. Eliot's writings and poetry. To her surprise, she discovers Eliot, a social and political conservative with strong religious prescriptions for cultural improvement, to be a less than passionate eugenics supporter. In Chapter 3, the writings of the avant-garde feminist writer Gertrude Stein are explored. Stein registered a feminist protest against conventional literary and medical techniques, but she also perpetuated quite conventional racist portraits of African Americans. English examines Stein's writings in the context of not only eugenics but also of the battle between obstetrics and midwifery that was being waged at the time. English contends there is an undercurrent of anxiety regarding the fecundity of the immigrant woman in America in Stein's writings.

The final two chapters contrast writings by New Negro female playwrights and by white eugenic field workers. In Chapter 4, the antilynching plays of Angelina Weld Grimke and others criticize eugenic ideology. English notes that in Grimke's 1916 play, *Rachel*, for example, "Lynching represents, then, a most unnatural form of selection, one designed to reinforce white supremacy and sustain black powerlessness, regardless of the quality and education of either whites or blacks" (p. 125). Indeed, Grimke's dramas and those by Georgia Douglas Johnson and Mary Burrill challenged not only racism but also an environment that selected against New Negro women. In contrast, English is particularly critical of the white, female eugenic field workers. Chapter 5 chronicles their thoughts in written documentation located in the Eugenics Record Office in Cold Spring Harbor, New York. These field workers' pens offer a disturbing glimpse into not only the ideology but also the actual practice of eugenics. Those persons deemed "defective" or dysgenic were often forcibly sterilized based on the recommendation of these laywomen.

In the conclusion, English warns against judging the Progressive Era, modernism, and the Harlem Renaissance by contemporary standards. We in the twenty-first century realize that eugenic thinking led directly to one of the greatest atrocities of modern time, the Holocaust. Since the mid-1940s, the word "eugenics" carries the connotation of disdain and immorality, but the wrongness of eugenic thinking was not apparent to the American writers of the 1920s.

In her analysis of texts by a myriad of authors, English clearly demonstrates that the social ideology of eugenics knew no class, gender, or race boundaries. This gives weight to her argument of the pervasiveness of eugenic thinking in American society in the early twentieth century. English not only references the aforementioned authors, but she also includes contemporary literary scholars of modernism and the Harlem Renaissance. Through the critiques of these scholars, the reader is aided in deciphering the often difficult literary styles of Eliot, Stein, DuBois, and the female New Negro playwrights.

This book is a welcome addition to the growing body of work that addresses eugenic ideology. English's unique methodology and literary background bring a refreshing perspective. The social commentary she raises is particularly pertinent in today's environment. Most compelling is English's link of historical thought to practices today, such as genetic engineering, fertility enhancement and control, and legislation promoting or discouraging family growth. She argues that these are contemporary equivalents of eugenics.

Unnatural Selections captures the profound effect eugenic thinking had on modern literature and society. In the 1920s, eugenics was equated with social uplift and progressiveness.

Now, eugenics carries a stigma often associated with forced sterilization and mass exter-
mination. This book begs the questions: How will today's marvels of medical and social
science be interpreted by future generations, and how will contemporary authors, po-
ets, playwrights, and activists write our story? These are some of the social and ethical
questions this book may evoke in its readers. Anyone with an interest in history, literature,
medicine, social policy, women's studies, or African-American studies will find this book
intriguing.

MOLLIE K. HANLON, RN, BSN, CCRN
Major, Army Nurse Corps
Graduate Student
Purdue University School of Nursing
West Lafayette, IN 47907

1. Gail Bederman, *Manliness and Civilization: A Cultural History of Gender and Race in the United
States, 1880–1917* (Chicago: University of Chicago Press, 1995).

Motherhood in Bondage

By Margaret Sanger; foreword by Margaret Marsh
(Columbus: Ohio State University Press, 2000) (472 pages; $57.95 cloth;
$19.95 paper)

Motherhood in Bondage, printed in 1928 and recently re-released by The Ohio State University Press, was one of Margaret Sanger's tomes arguing for women's right to contraceptive
care. Originally trained as a nurse, Sanger recognized the pressing necessity of securing safe,
reliable birth control methods for women of all social classes. She devoted her life and career
to this mission and was once jailed for violating interstate obscenity laws. Through books,
pamphlets, speeches, and court battles, she became the most famous birth control advocate
of the twentieth century. With *Motherhood*, Sanger attempted to harness the first-person
accounts of suffering mothers to convince the public to lobby in favor of the birth control
movement.
    The timeless relevance of the book's subject matter cannot be denied. During the past
two years, U.S. Food and Drug Administration hearings, Senate examinations of Supreme
Court nominees, and discussions in the lay media and professional journals prove the
contemporary resonance of the politics of motherhood and fertility. Despite this topicality,
however, *Motherhood* rings surprisingly hollow. Both politically and emotionally unaffecting,
the volume, a compilation of 470 letters received by Sanger from women nationwide, reads as
repetitive and flat. Although certain letters are engaging and effectively crystallize women's
struggles, the redundancy of the stories, combined with the sheer volume (*Motherhood*
contains an exhausting 400 pages of letter excerpts), nearly inures the reader to their impact.
The stories impress with the desperation of the women's tone and of their circumstances;
however, Sanger's first and more well-known book, *Woman and the New Race*, provides a
more concise, articulate, and readable exploration of the topic.

Sanger's introduction, in which she lays out the themes and goals of the book, may be the most affecting and readable part of *Motherhood in Bondage*. Each chapter begins with a brief introduction reiterating her argumentative stance and summarizing the missives. The letter excerpts follow, grouped thematically into such chapters as "Girl Mothers" and "Doctor Warns – But Does Not Tell." The choppily edited letters narrate what Sanger terms the "bondage of enforced maternity" (p. xlv). One of the most notable aspects of the women's experiences tends to be the number of pregnancies. One thirty-one-year-old woman writes that she is "the mother of eight living children, one baby dead and a three months miscarriage" (p. 15). Nearly all of the women live in extreme poverty, with little health care and no access to birth control. The scourges of their impoverished status compound inextricably their "enforced maternity."

As a nod to the eugenics movement, popular at the time, Sanger describes many of the women as "biologically 'unfit'" (p. 102) and decries the "disastrous folly of bringing defective children into the world" (p. 101). The letter writers themselves declare their unfitness for motherhood, due to a variety of physical, mental, and social conditions. The women argue Sanger's case that they ought to be able to control their own fertility, especially if potential children would be endangered by genetic conditions, inadequate nutrition, or other strained resources.

By 1928, when this book was published, Sanger had distanced herself from the anarchists and socialists who were the core of her support at the outset of her campaign. *Motherhood in Bondage* was part of her campaign to appeal to a broader audience, including lay readers, supporters of eugenics, and the medical community. Although some allies criticized her abandonment of radicalism, others accepted this more centrist position and continued to support her and the birth control cause. Perhaps Sanger's pragmatism and her willingness to compromise can help inform present debates about abortion, stem cell research, and other "hot button" issues that continually divide voters and commentators.

The dire tone of many letters does present a compelling explanation for Sanger's fervor and for her insistence on this particular book structure. One letter writer implores, "I hope to hear from you in the near future as you are my last deliverer but death" (p. 64). No reader could neglect the sadness of these women's experience and the heavy impact of poverty, loneliness, and poor health on their lives. Sanger correctly claims that "the story of motherhood in bondage is, by and large, the same story – the same pattern of pain, except here producing the same cry for deliverance" (p. xlvi). *Motherhood* is notable in its use of poor women as feminist voices. A common critique of both first- and second-wave feminists is their neglect of nonwealthy, uneducated women. This work contradicts this notion. Indeed, the fact that many of the letter writers cite *Woman and the New Race* speaks to the broad appeal of Sanger's message.

Historian Margaret Marsh has written a concise and informative foreword summarizing the life and career of Margaret Sanger and placing this volume in its historical context. For anyone interested in the history of birth control or of Sanger herself, the foreword may be impetus enough to pick up the book. The book also illustrates the less strident tone that Sanger took in her later years and provides some insight into her methods. However, the book's biased selection and editing processes limits use of the letters themselves as primary documents.

Motherhood in Bondage did not sell well at its first release, but as Marsh explains, "its sad stories were not comfortable reading for the prosperous middle-class, book-buying public at the time" (p. xxxv). For historians or practitioners of women's health care, the stories may not be novel or enlightening but may serve as confirmation of the necessity of preserving and encouraging the voices and rights of women.

Lisa Stern Slifka, RN
MSN Candidate
Yale University School of Nursing
New Haven, CT 06536

Compassion and Competence: Nursing in Mandatory Palestine, 1918–1948 חמלה וירע ראשית מקצוע הסיעור בארץ ישראל

By Nira Bartal
(Jerusalem: Yard Izhak Ben-Zvi, 2005) (Hebrew, 444 pages; 98 NIS; $21 cloth)

Compassion and Competence is a comprehensive and thorough overview of the development of nursing in Mandatory Palestine from 1918 to 1948. The accounts of nursing during those years, as argued by Nira Bartal, have shaped the profession of the modern Hebrew and then Israeli nurse, as well as the development of nursing as a profession in this region. It should also be seen within the global context of the changes that shaped the nursing profession. In her outstanding analysis, Bartal discusses topics such as the study of nursing history, the creation and progress of nursing education, nursing as a feminine domain, and the specific story of the Hadassah School of Nursing in Jerusalem.

This historical analysis covers various periods that are all considered to be during the time of the British Mandate in Palestine. The first part focuses on the years between 1918 and 1933 when American nurses came to join Hadassah with a mission to prepare a structure and foundation that would tackle the problem of poor public health in Palestine. These Zionist Jewish Hadassah nurses helped define nursing and lay a basis for educating the former "noneducated" nurses to become professionals in their own territory and community settings. The more traditional Florence Nightingale concept of nursing dominated this period. The second part is devoted to the years 1933 to 1948, until the establishment of the State of Israel, which is characterized by the professional and academic development of nursing, as well as by the design of a curriculum to train nurses for future work. It should be emphasized that influences from abroad came both from British nursing, which influenced more the formal and political status of nursing, and from the American system, which was clinically advanced and more academic.

Bartal has conducted extensive research, which includes archival work, analysis of historical documents, and hours of interviews of nursing figures who led the field and who left a mark in the profession's history. Her descriptions of the aspects that influenced nursing and the role of nursing, then, are therefore presented through the eyes of influential women such as Henrietta Zold, Shulamit Kantor, and others. Moreover, Bartal provides the reader with an insight into the everyday life of nursing teachers and students at the time, as well as the general poor and problematic hospital environments that characterized those years. Conditions related to accommodation and general life of the students are portrayed with stories that give flair to her critical historical analysis. Many anecdotes are related to the relationship between the medical profession and the growing development of nursing as a paramedical profession. The hospital's structure and the health care situation of these years are the background stage for Bartal's fascinating performance. The inclusion of many pictures also helps the reader comprehend the context of the stories.

Compassion and Competence is a feminine story of women's immigration to Israel, a story of women wanting to have a profession, and a story of the creation of the State of Israel. However, beyond all of this, it highlights the struggle of nursing in its fight to gain professional and academic credibility. This is a book that every nurse should read in order to understand how nursing has become what it is today and the history of its origins. Its global implications, however, are the real message, with a specific local influence. The book can be of interest to nurses both in America and in Taiwan, each country having its own professional history with similar motives. It would have been interesting to see a continuation of this particular story in terms of the status of nursing once the State of Israel was created and the influence of nursing from abroad on this development.

Bartal leaves the reader with many questions as to how this story of courage and devotion has shaped the Israeli nurse of today, who lives within a professional environment that, to her, is in many respects an unquestionable norm. How is the nursing student of previous times, who lived a rigorous dorm life with strict uniform codes and no time for social interactions and cross-gender life, similar and different from the modern student who wears white jeans to work, may live in a rented flat, and studies in a more democratic environment?

ILANA KADMON, RN, PHD
Hadassah and the Hebrew University School of Nursing
P.O. Box 12000
Jerusalem 91120
Israel

Care to Remember: Nursing and Midwifery in Ireland
Edited by Gerard M. Fealy
(Douglas Village, Cork, Ireland: Mercier Press, 2005) (224 pages; €20.00 paper)

Historians, write Martha Howell and Walter Prevenier in *From Reliable Sources*, do not discover the past. Rather, they create it. They choose the events, the ideas, the people, or the institutions they think embody an important piece of the past. They then decide what about them is important to know. Finally, they construct interpretations responsibly, with care, and with a high degree of self-consciousness about the reasons behind their particular choices and decisions.[1] The essays presented in *Care to Remember: Nursing and Midwifery in Ireland* deserve a reading in their own right as examples of just such reflexive history: they represent the best and the most recent research of a productive and diverse group of clinical and academic scholars centered in and around University College Dublin. But it is as a whole that we see the strength and the importance of *Care to Remember*. This collection of essays marks, I believe, the beginning of a new Irish history of nursing and midwifery: in the choice of topics, in the focused stories, and in the careful and thoughtful construction of interpretations, we see the outlines of a self-confident history for a self-confident profession in a self-confident nation.

The five essays in Part 1 of *Care to Remember* lay out the contextual background for the new nursing and midwifery history by reflecting on the issues raised by past images of nursing and midwifery in Ireland. As Gerard M. Fealy and Malcolm Newby point out in "Through the Lens," the construction of particular images has long been a part of Irish culture. Following Irish independence in 1922, for example, Éamon de Valera, Ireland's first president, believed the country's image should be that of a romantic pastoralism: an idyllic, self-sufficient, and hardy agrarian culture of good Catholics uncorrupted by foreign cultural influences. But, the construction of health care images, as Fealy argues in another essay with Mary O'Doherty, were the almost exclusive purview of amateur physician historians who loved to tell stereotypical stories of the drunk and incompetent untrained nurse, the oppressed probationer, the self-effacing nun, the powerful ward sister, the loyal and devoted nurse, and the firm but always fair matron.

Not surprisingly, as Margaret Pearl Tracy points out in "Invisible Nursing," the important contributions of real flesh-and-blood nurses remained unseen: the traditions of the "silent knowledge" of the Catholic nursing orders hushed nursing's voice on the wards, in the public debate, and in the articulation of health care policy. But, the country's 1973 entry into the European Economic Union forever changed the political, economic, social, educational, and clinical landscape. Ireland now looked aggressively outward, and, in 1979 and again in 1991, the Irish Nursing Board (An Bord Altranais) implemented a number of European directives on the training of nurses. The foundations of the older apprentice system crumbled as the hours devoted to classroom learning increased and the range of clinical experiences broadened. This system finally ended forever in 2002. Irish nursing, with the strong support of the Irish state, found its voice. Now, a four-year university degree is the only route of entry into Irish nursing practice.

Still, as Martin McNamara explains in "Dr. Nightingale, I Presume?," the admittedly "massive social experiment" (p. 54) that inalterably links Irish nursing and higher education has simultaneously generated a public debate that ranges from support to unease to downright disdain. His historical analysis of the language in and through which this debate has been conducted reveals a set of recurring images and metaphors remarkably reminiscent of those of the late nineteenth and early twentieth centuries. The concept of the educated nurse remains enduringly problematic, and Irish nurses today must confront the fear that they are "too posh to wash." Moreover, as Peter Nolan emphasizes in "Caring, Past and Present," they must confront such fears within an increasingly strained and understaffed health care system.

How might Irish nurses understand and appreciate such historic (although not unproblematic) accomplishments? How might they answer their detractors and sustain (and even broaden) their professional initiatives? The historians' answers can be found in Part 2 of Care to Remember. Here, we have historians giving Irish nurses new stories: stories of nurses who do not fear foreign influences, but embrace them; stories of institutions embedded in Catholic traditions, but keen to acknowledge the social and economic power of new secular (or, at least, nonsectarian) organizations; and, in the end, stories of a people and a profession tightly tied to the grand international nursing project that we know as the invention of modern nursing.

Siobhan Horgan-Ryan, for example, in "Irish Military Nursing in the Great War," creates a past in which the best educated of Irish nurses, like their sisters in Australia, the United States, Great Britain, and Canada, proved their worth through service to their country. Irish nurses, in fact, joined Queen Alexandra's Imperial Military Nursing Service Reserve in far greater numbers than previously recognized; and they did so even after the 1916 Easter Sunday Rebellion against Great Britain.

Ann Wickham, in her study of the early years of district nursing in late-nineteenth- and early-twentieth-century Ireland, creates another past in which the traditions of Catholic charity and Protestant philanthropy find some common cause in support of the work of Queen Victoria's Jubilee Institute for Nurses (QVJIN), an initiative that brought trained nurses into the homes of the sick poor.[2] As Wickham points out, the advent of the QVJIN in Ireland coincided with the introduction of lay nurse training by the major Catholic nursing orders. Although problems remained, tensions often ran high, and the QVJIN remained committed to sending nurses of similar denominations to areas with specific denominational majorities. The emphasis on shared training and skills meant that the work of Catholic Queen's nurses matched that of their Protestant sisters.

Such work is the focus of Therese Meehan's oral history of Mary Quinn, a Catholic QVJIN nurse supported by the Lady Dudley Nursing Scheme, which brought women trained as nurses and midwives to towns and villages too poor to support a QVJIN on their own. In Meehan's telling, Quinn's practice in the Galway village of An Cheathrú Rua in the late 1930s serves as a model for contemporary nursing practice. For Meehan, Quinn's ability, thoughtfulness, and propensity for independent thought and judgment stands as the strongest historical rebuttal to those who believe that excellence in practice, intellectual enthusiasm, and strong faith are mutually exclusive.

Declan Devane and Jo Murphy-Lawless, in their close readings of seminal texts on childbirth, and Ann McMahon, in her story of the role of the Royal College of Physicians of Ireland in promoting regulated midwifery practice, tell stories that more closely link Irish experiences of increasing medical and scientific authority with that of other European countries. But Ann Sheridan, in her study of Irish psychiatric nurses in the 1950s, tells a story about the limits of just such authority. Here, de Valera's image of idyllic, self-sufficient, and hardy Catholics uncorrupted by foreign cultural influences held full sway. In part, the limited economic resources of the new Irish Free State meant prioritizing needs. Initiatives that improved the general health and living standards of its people – that would create and maintain just such hardy Catholics – took precedence. The mentally ill had no constituency that might advance its cause. The Catholic Church hierarchy held firm in its antipathy to the notions of behavioralism, psychoanalysis, and psychodynamic psychotherapy that were transforming psychiatry and psychiatric nursing in Europe and the United States.

Marie Carney's "Nurses as Managers" concludes the histories in *Care to Remember*, telling the stories of Catholic and secular nursing leaders throughout recent Irish history. In all, there are many stories told, and many that remain. Irish nurses still need stories that tell, for example, what it was like being a woman in a Catholic and conservative country, or stories that more deeply explore the tensions between religious and secular impulses in nursing. But, for now, Irish nurses are well served by historians who are creating new meanings and memories for a new generation of professionals.

PATRICIA D'ANTONIO, RN, PhD, FAAN
Adjunct Associate Professor of Nursing
Barbara Bates Center for the Study of the History of Nursing
University of Pennsylvania
Philadelphia, PA 19104

1. Martha Howell and Walter Prevenier, *From Reliable Sources: An Introduction to Historical Methods* (Ithaca and London: Cornell University Press, 2001): 1, 148.
2. The QVJIN, dedicated to providing skilled nursing to the sick poor in their own homes, had been established in honor of the Queen in London in 1887; and, by 1890, it had established local committees in both Edinburgh and Dublin. Ireland was seen as particularly problematic: in the early twentieth century, its capital city of Dublin had the fifth highest death rate in the world, the rural poor of the West fared little better, and Catholic religious leaders wanted their own separate system of district nurses.

On All Frontiers: Four Centuries of Canadian Nursing

Edited by Christina Bates, Dianne Dodd, and Nicole Rousseau
(Ottawa, Ontario, Canada: University of Ottawa Press, 2005) (248 pages; $50.00 paper). Also issued in French under the title *Sans Frontières: Quatre Siècles de Soins Infirmiers Canadiens*

The publication of *On All Frontiers* marks the third stage of an ambitious joint venture among the Canadian Nurses Association, the Canadian Museum of Civilization, the Canadian War Museum, and Library and Archives Canada to bring together and make accessible important nursing collections in Canada. Preceded by the creation of the Canadian Nursing History Collection and the development of a major exhibition on nursing history, *On All Frontiers* was envisioned as a comprehensive history for both nursing historians and the general reader. Although its coffee-table dimensions, rich archival illustrations, and numerous vignettes will undoubtedly appeal to a broad audience, the front cover does not do justice to the content, nor is the size and binding type conducive to easy reading. Instead, its strength lies in the depth of analysis demonstrated by the contributing authors – an impressive collection of recognized scholars of Canadian nursing history.

   On All Frontiers is the first comprehensive book on Canadian nursing history since John Gibbon's *Three Centuries of Canadian Nursing* was published in 1947. Although others have looked at the development of Canadian nursing after 1870 in English Canada (e.g., Kathryn McPherson's *Bedside Matters: The Transformation of Canadian Nursing*, 1996; Diana Mansell's *Forging the Future: A History of Nursing in Canada*, 2004), this study is distinctive in the variety of subjects covered, including attention to – and comparison of – the unique and overlapping trajectories of English and French Canadian nursing history across the centuries. Although certain key areas of Canadian nursing history are under-represented or overlooked (e.g., mental health nursing, international and missionary nursing, graduate nursing education, aboriginal nursing), *On All Frontiers* covers a surprising range of nursing roles, effectively portraying Canadian nursing as intriguing, contentious, and complex.

   Organized around the central theme of nurses as ubiquitous and influential participants in the development of Canada, *On All Frontiers* is divided into fourteen chapters clustered under categories of "place" – that is, home, hospital, community, frontier, battlefield, classroom, boardroom, and picket line. By choosing place rather than time as the organizing framework, the editors created a unique opportunity for contributing scholars to explore the interplay among religion, politics, gender, culture, nation, and region. Using primary data, *On All Frontiers* successfully advances new and particular understandings of Canadian history without losing sight of broader evolutionary patterns; it is both compelling and rigorous. Nurses emerge as essential players in the evolution of a country now defined by its commitment to a universal health care system, accessible to all Canadians.

As a nurse historian and educator, I was pleased to have many gaps in my own understanding of Canadian history filled in and contextualized. For example, Pauline Paul identifies the widespread influence of French Catholic nuns on organized nursing after 1760, a movement that led to the development of hospitals in all major cities in western Canada. Kathryn McPherson explores the influence of Nightingale on the development of the modern hospital after 1870, concluding that Canadian hospitals and training schools were actually a hybrid of the Nightingale system, where administrative authority and control over nursing education as envisioned by Nightingale was never achieved. Lynn Kirkwood argues that training schools in English Canada after 1874 emerged as practical means to an end of improving hospital organization and service and were not intended to further the cause of higher learning – a legacy that has subtly undermined university education in Canada ever since.

Most fascinating is the central argument that nurses, through their response to many types of calls (e.g., midwives, district nurses, political activists, military nurses), have contributed to the shaping of a nation. Dianne Dodd, Jayne Elliot, and Nicole Rousseau provide a poignant example of this in their chapter on outpost nurses. They conclude that ventures to support small and remote communities reinforced a sense of public entitlement to health care, increasing pressure for state funding.

On All Frontiers is a landmark text. I strongly recommend it as an essential resource for nursing educators and any scholars interested in nursing, labor, women's, and Canadian history.

SONYA GRYPMA, RN, PhD
SSHRC Postdoctoral Research Fellow
University of British Columbia
Assistant Professor
School of Health Sciences
University of Lethbridge
Lethbridge, AB T1K 3M4 Canada

"Must We All Die?": Alaska's Enduring Struggle with Tuberculosis

By Robert Fortuine

(Fairbanks: University of Alaska Press, 2005) (304 pages; $39.95 cloth)

Tuberculosis has been with humans for thousands of years, although its origins are not clear. It is a serious, chronic, infectious disease that if left untreated can lead to death and disability. Although the occurrence of tuberculosis is in decline in the United States, the disease is still a major public health threat worldwide. The rising global incidence of tuberculosis in recent years, due mainly to the HIV/AIDS epidemic, gives *"Must We All Die?"* a compelling and immediate importance.

This book tells the story of tuberculosis in Alaska, where the disease nearly decimated the Native American population prior to World War II, a time when public health efforts to combat tuberculosis became more effective. This book also tells the story of those efforts by dedicated public health officials and workers to develop a system to research, prevent, and treat tuberculosis despite scarce financial resources and political and bureaucratic obstacles. Organizational history comprises a large portion of *"Must We All Die?"*. It is described in great detail and includes such organizations as the Bureau of Education, the Office of Indian Affairs, the Alaska Tuberculosis Association, the Alaska Native Service, the Territorial Health Department, and the Alaska Health Department. The roles of significant players within these organizations are highlighted throughout.

The book is organized by themes and follows a chronological development. However, the chronology is difficult to follow in that it is described within each chapter as opposed to throughout the entire book. It is well referenced from numerous sources, both primary and secondary. Interesting quotes from physicians, nurses, and public health workers are interspersed throughout the book to give it a rich context.

Robert Fortuine consistently and clearly uses public health data to demonstrate the lack of interest in and funding for public health initiatives to combat tuberculosis in Alaskan Natives. However, he reserves comment on the racial underpinnings of this neglect, relying instead on just the factual data. One example of racism was the practice of Alaskan officials to couch efforts toward tuberculosis control and treatment in Alaskan Natives in terms of protecting the white population. The similarities between the present-day scourge and neglect of tuberculosis in vulnerable populations globally and in Africa, in particular, are evident to the reader, but the text provides little analysis.

The voice of nurses, some named and others not, are prominent throughout this story of the Alaskan battle against tuberculosis. Prior to the discovery of modern drug therapy to treat tuberculosis, the frontline battle involved the public health initiatives of personal and village cleanliness, control of spitting, and ventilation. One nurse, Ada J. Van Vranken, reported the dangers of "promiscuous spitting" (p. 32), the practice of spitting onto the floor in crowded living units. Public health nurses played an important role in health education and promotion, although the imposition of Western values regarding sanitation and cleanliness is evident.

The lived experiences of the Native American patients in sanatoriums are painstakingly detailed in an appendix, which, in this reviewers' view, should have been a central chapter of the book rather than an afterthought to the body of the text. In the 1940s, tuberculosis sanatorium beds were in short supply, and the waiting period for beds could be up to two years. Once a bed became available, an Alaskan Native who had been diagnosed with tuberculosis would be removed from his or her village and flown hundreds of miles from home for treatment where the chance of recovery was uncertain. These patients were removed suddenly and usually alone to a strange location in an unfamiliar culture to be placed on strict bed rest. At the same time, the structure and activity of sanatorium life was rigid. The Native Alaskans were isolated in a strange land where they did not speak the language and often faced a solitary death away from family.

As a result of modern drug treatment for tuberculosis in the 1950s, mortality from the disease in Alaska markedly declined. However, the occurrence and incidence rates continue to be significantly higher for Native Alaskans than whites through 2002 (as reported in the book). The book ends on a positive note, with an endearing story of Robert Sam, an Alaskan Native who worked to return the remains of tuberculosis victims to their families for burial. These patients had been interred on Japonski Island between 1947 and 1966 in bunkers after dying in sanatoriums because of a lack of funds to return their remains to their families. Through the efforts of Mr. Sam and numerous individuals and agencies, many family members were able to grieve and return the remains of their loved ones to their homes for burial. This story serves as an example of the finest qualities of Alaska's conflict with tuberculosis.

"Must We All Die?" provides important historical documentation about tuberculosis in Alaska, its effect on the Native Alaskans and the men and women who worked tirelessly to combat it, and the obstacles they encountered. Historians of nursing and medicine will find it useful.

MARJORIE L. PORTER, RN, EdD
Associate Professor
University of Indianapolis
Indianapolis, IN 46227

Pain and Profits: The History of the Headache and Its Remedies in America
By Jan R. McTavish
(New Brunswick, NJ: Rutgers University Press, 2004) (239 pages; $23.95 paper)

For most of humans' existence, headaches posed a perplexing and, in general, resistant problem for patients who experienced them and medical practitioners who were called on for treatment. As Jan R. McTavish points out in *Pain and Profits: The History of the Headache and Its Remedies in America*, the availability of safe, effective remedies with which to treat headaches is a relatively recent phenomenon. In this well-written and interesting work,

McTavish uses the headache and its treatment to examine not only the history of headache relief but also the complex interrelationships among number of different interest groups, including physicians, patients, the drug industry, advertising agencies, and the government, as science devised solutions for the ordinary headache. As might be expected, given the name of the book, profits played a major role in headache treatment. Intertwined within this multifaceted story is a compelling discussion of control over medical practice, treatment choice, the rise of the modern headache relief industry, and the emergence of government regulation of prescripting practices. Some interesting conclusions on medical control over everyday treatment regimens are also drawn.

Arranging the book in chronological order, McTavish recounts that few effective headache remedies existed before the twentieth century. This situation changed dramatically in the late nineteenth century with the introduction of synthetic drugs into the market. Designed as antipyretics and produced predominantly by the German chemical industry expanding into the lucrative pharmaceutical business, the original synthetic drugs reduced fevers and possessed the added benefit of conferring significant pain relief. Developed in 1899 by the Bayer Company, aspirin became the classic ideal of a synthetic drug. It was inexpensive, fast-acting, specific, and had relatively few serious side effects. In McTavish's words, headaches had finally "met their match" (p. 153).

Drug and pharmaceutical companies figure prominently in this story. The nineteenth-century American drug industry divided into two camps: the "ethical" firms, dedicated to producing standardized, unadulterated products; and the patent drug companies and nostrum makers that offered patent medicines of dubious contents and worth. This division resulted in a highly competitive pharmaceutical market. Nostrum and patent medicine makers further separated themselves from the "ethicals" by advertising directly and vigorously to the general public. Ethical drug companies looked down on this practice and limited their advertising to physicians, thus forging a bond between the presumably more scientific approach of contemporary medicine and pharmaceutical interests.

The advent of synthetic drugs created numerous problems for drug companies, pharmacists, and physicians because synthetics possessed several characteristics generally associated with patent medicines. They were prepackaged, initially as powders and later in pill form, and patented; and their contents were predetermined to treat specific maladies. Synthetic pain relievers robbed regular physicians and pharmacists of the valued tradition, which dictated that the physician compose prescriptions based on careful medical analysis of the patient's symptoms and that the pharmacist compound these prescriptions based on a scientific knowledge of the ingredients. The use of easily remembered trademark names for synthetic drugs challenged power relationships between physicians and patients, pharmacists and physicians, and patients and pharmacists by allowing patients to go to a pharmacy to request, perhaps even to demand, certain drugs for minor aches and pains.

Large drug companies gained significant financial profits from marketing effective headache relief. Highlighted in two detailed chapters are the efforts of the Bayer Company, a German concern, to aggressively protect its patent and trademark rights first for its antipyretic product, phenacetin, and later for aspirin. After the U.S. government confiscated the American branch of Bayer during World War I, its successor, Sterling Products, a former nostrum maker, continued to defend but ultimately lost the trademark rights to the name aspirin, by then a best-selling headache relief. The name aspirin entered the public domain and escaped regulation as a prescription-only medication. This ensured that average individuals seeking pain relief could obtain effective products on their own without the intervention of professional medical or pharmaceutical help.

McTavish ends the story with a discussion of twentieth-century efforts to define and pinpoint the cause of headaches, an effort no more successful than earlier ones at identifying why headaches occur. With the exception of migraines, determining the underlying pathology of headaches continues to baffle medical science. As McTavish notes, however, most headache sufferers consider the availability of fast, effective, inexpensive pain relief more important than knowing why they developed the pain in the first place. The author concludes that patients continue to be able to maintain significant authority over their medical affairs, at least as far as headache treatment goes.

This book offers a thoughtful and detailed analysis of the challenges ordinary, mundane ailments posed for health care practitioners, medical science, and patients. McTavish unravels the active role the drug trade took in providing accessible pain relief and reveals the complex relationships existing among drug companies, physicians, and patients. Overall, this book is an intriguing read that makes a significant contribution to our understanding of how medical science and patients negotiated acceptable solutions to the occurrence of everyday aches and pains.

JEAN C. WHELAN, PhD, RN
Assistant Adjunct Professor of Nursing
Barbara Bates Center for the Study of the History of Nursing
University of Pennsylvania
Philadelphia, PA 19104

Choice and Coercion: Birth Control, Sterilization, and Abortion in Public Health and Welfare

By Johanna Schoen
(Chapel Hill: University of North Carolina Press, 2005) (352 pages; $59.95 cloth, $19.95 paper)

In *Choice and Coercion*, Johanna Schoen highlights the double-edged nature of reproductive technologies: "they could extend reproductive control to women, or they could be used to control women's reproduction" (p. 3). Although Schoen's focus is on the historical development of the role of sterilization, abortion, and other reproductive technologies in public health and welfare policies, her words capture the controversy facing policy makers and citizens in the United States today. Indeed, the book's publication is aptly timed given the recent vacancies on the U.S. Supreme Court, which could affect women's reproductive rights.

Those seeking a better understanding of the current controversy would do well by reading *Choice and Coercion* because it is a thoroughly researched and well-written contribution to the study of reproductive health. In analyzing birth control, sterilization, and abortion policy making in the twentieth century, the author draws from an impressive collection of manuscripts, interviews, newspapers, periodicals, books, articles, and dissertations. Most important, Schoen reviewed 8,000 sterilization petitions dating from 1934 to 1966 and eventually obtained access to the minutes from meetings of the Eugenics Board that enabled her to tell the stories of women, families, physicians, and social workers involved with family planning during this time. Her work helps show how birth control, sterilization, and abortion could be either liberating or controlling, according to society's beliefs about race and gender at the time. She specifically focuses on North Carolina's reproductive health care system during the early to mid-twentieth century, not because it is an anomaly but because it resembled policy creation and implementation in other places in the United States and abroad. In her comparison of policies in North Carolina to situations in Puerto Rico and India, Schoen takes her study to the international level. She writes, "Economic underdevelopment, poverty, perceived overpopulation, and a demographic otherness" made portions of the United States, Puerto Rico, and India all "ripe for the scientific and sexual experiments of philanthropy" (p. 8).

To examine this experimentation and its social, political, and economic effects, the author divides the book into four chapters, each of which builds on the tension between women's control over their own reproduction and the power of health professionals and policy makers to control population. The book closes with an eye-opening epilogue containing a critique of current sterilization reparation measures.

The first chapter provides an historical account of birth control services in North Carolina, South Carolina, and Tennessee for poor white and black populations, emphasizing the "lack of a coherent delivery system" and the resulting "patchwork of services of uneven quality" (p. 24). Many rural women had little or no access to birth control services but were frequently used in contraceptive field trials and experiments. A central character in the chapter is Nina Hillard, a birth control nurse paid by philanthropist Clarence Gamble. Hillard often found herself in conflict with the rigid research protocols as she empathized with her clients' desires for one form of contraception over another. This chapter concludes by introducing the irony in the government's preference, after World War II, for family planning and population control to lower health care costs and welfare dependency, while limiting women's access to the method.

In Chapter 2, Schoen examines the politics of sterilization through the creative use of a eugenics poem written by Boston philanthropist and birth control activist, Clarence Gamble, in the mid-1940s. The poem not only echoes popular sentiment of the time by celebrating eugenics, but it also provides a rich starting point to discuss the different aspects of sterilization. In fact, Schoen uses verses from the poem to introduce each section of the chapter. For example, in an outline of the criteria used for sterilizations, the subheading "Eugenic Science and the Making of Eugenic Sterilization Laws" is accompanied by the stanza, "*Once there was a MORON, that means/ A person who wasn't very bright./ He couldn't add figures/ Or make change/ Or do many things/ An ordinary man does*" (p. 81). Typical criteria used to justify sterilization were mental disease, feeblemindedness, poverty, welfare dependency, alcoholism, mental illness, and promiscuity. The subjective nature of the criteria makes it easy to see how the poor were at a disadvantage because they were "more likely than others to be targeted for involuntary sterilization, but they were also disproportionately denied access to voluntary sterilization" (p. 138). Here, the theme of choice (poor women's agency) or coercion (control over their reproduction) was especially evident. At the same time, a state-sponsored Eugenics Board was one of the few resources that poor or minority women could use if they wanted greater reproductive control.

The main focus of Chapter 3 is the political and social context surrounding abortion in the twentieth century. Competing definitions of abortion (elective, therapeutic, and eugenic) were integral parts of the abortion controversy. Before *Roe v. Wade* in 1973, women who had little access to contraception often sought abortions to prevent impoverished circumstances from getting worse. However, because abortion was illegal, it was hard to find physicians who would agree to perform them. Thus, women had to find a willing doctor, pay high prices for services, and sometimes agree to sterilization before the physician would perform the abortion. Often, women found loopholes (usually linguistic in nature) to obtain what they wanted. For example, just as some women lied and said that they were "feebleminded" in order to be sterilized as a form of family planning, women also "admitted" to being mentally ill in order to get abortions.

The theme of control versus agency continues in the fourth chapter, which examines family planning in an international setting during a time when scientists were beginning to shift their focus from individual eugenics to large-scale population management. To help readers remain mindful of the close link between local policies and global politics, Schoen incorporates international comparisons. This chapter reveals similarities rather than differences in reproductive control rhetoric used by government officials from Puerto Rico, India, and the United States. All three nations feared that government assistance might create a "permanent relief class" and thus withheld services, including reproductive health care, from their citizens (p. 236). Along with the deprivation of basic services, these underserved populations became the targets of medical testing because they were "more pliable, and less likely to ask questions," among other reasons (p. 239).

The epilogue to *Choice and Coercion* is one of the most provocative sections of the book and includes criticism of government public apologies for sterilization. In February 2003, the North Carolina governor publicly apologized to the victims of sterilization and formed a special commission to consider providing restitution. Schoen argues, however, that apologies tended to cut off further discussions; and, in some cases, certain states took them as a sign to close or destroy records. She urges the reader to reconsider the significance we attribute to official apologies and to examine what will actually create lasting change in women's lives. As an activist, Schoen felt responsible to educate the public about the wrong that had been done and to give that history the recognition it deserved. In addition, the book's academic focus can be of use in educating students in the history of women, nursing, medicine, and health policy.

REBEKAH FOX
PhD Student, Communication/Rhetorical Studies
Purdue University
West Lafayette, IN 47907

Dying to Be Beautiful: The Fight for Safe Cosmetics

By Gwen Kay

(Columbus: The Ohio State University Press, 2005) (224 pages; $64.95 cloth, $22.95 paper)

Dying to Be Beautiful: The Fight for Safe Cosmetics is part of a series on *Women, Gender, and Health,* edited by Susan L. Smith and Nancy Tomes. It was written by Gwen Kay, who is currently an Assistant Professor of History at the State University of New York at Oswego. Based on her dissertation research at Yale University, this book won a 2005 *AJN* Book of the Year Award. This well-researched work reviews the history of the regulation of cosmetics and assorted "beauty products" during the first half of the twentieth century. As such, it ties together several disparate strands: not only of political activism, notably of women, but also more broadly of an emerging consumer movement; the history of medicine; changing notions of beauty, femininity, and health; the associated products and industries spawned to meet these ideals; and the emergence of the corresponding need for federal regulation of some of these products and industries. This tying together of strands is both the book's strength and its weakness.

In the course of telling this story, Kay covers a wide variety of material to highlight how women, in particular, and consumers, in general, impact a product's success in the marketplace. In addition, she describes how various constituencies interact and ultimately contribute to the enactment of federal legislation. A wide variety of other issues affect this tale. For example, Kay integrates varying and changing notions of beauty, health, and cleanliness; the changing roles of women over the course of the first half of the twentieth century; and how women used cosmetics and beauty products to express and reflect these changing mores. The book also covers the history of cosmetics and the beauty industry; the impact of various pieces of legislation; and the interaction of the rising medical profession, especially dermatology, with the cosmetic and beauty industry, rooted in skin and hair care.

The book is organized into five chapters, with an introduction and a short epilogue. Chapter 1 focuses on the passage of the 1906 Pure Food and Drug Act. Kay documents the active role of women's organizations, specifically the Women's Christian Temperance Union and the General Federation of Women's Clubs, which worked to promote laws to protect consumers. These organizations relied on activism at the local level. Even after the passage of legislation in 1906, local chapters of these organizations were vigilant in ensuring adequate, prompt, and vigorous enforcement of the law. Kay notes that although beauty products were becoming mass-produced during this time, they escaped the scrutiny of the 1906 act.

In the second chapter, Kay focuses on the growth of the cosmetic market through the early 1930s. She nicely situates this in the context of increasing societal homogeneity and an emphasis on youth fostered by the rise of mass-circulated magazines and advertising. In addition, the increasing use of mass-produced beauty products fostered a variety of employment niches for women: door-to-door sales, cosmeticians, and beauty salon workers and owners. In the third chapter, the theme of activism is reprised. The rise of consumer groups replaced organizations exclusively focused on women, which had declined after the passage of woman's suffrage. These activists, along with physicians who treated the after effects of cosmetics run amok, expressed increased concerns regarding the cosmetic industry. The early 1930s was a time of increasing government regulation and involvement.

Chapters 4 and 5 revolve around the events leading up to the passage of the 1938 Food, Drug, and Cosmetics Act (effective June 1939) and the immediate aftermath. The 1938 law was an extensive revamping of the 1906 Pure Food and Drug Act. It passed, in part, due to activism of some unlikely bedfellows in the form of consumer groups, the medical profession, and women's organizations, all of whom testified before Congress. Years of careful lobbying by these groups over a five-year period, however, had not yielded success. Bogged down in interagency squabbling, it took the death of 114 people from "sulfanilamide elixir" to lead to eventual passage of the 1938 law. It empowered the U.S. Food and Drug Administration to seize unsafe products; and the agency, aided by alert physicians, aggressively pursued this policy.

In the epilogue, Kay makes note of the numerous and necessary revisions to the 1938 Food, Drug, and Cosmetics Act over time. She points out current issues related to the cosmetic industry, now affecting both men and women, such as hair implants and Botox injections. The bottom line remains the same: protecting the consumer. Kay argues that the story told in *Dying to Be Beautiful* "... demonstrates how everyday people on a local level contributed to a national policy shift" (p. 8). The financial interests of the manufacturers themselves also played a part in this story because safe products are equated, ultimately, with good business. Kay states, "... ultimately, although consumers can impact regulation and legislation on multiple levels, their real power is the marketplace, determining the success or failure of a product" (p. 8).

The book's many strengths I found also to be its weakness: a somewhat blurred focus. I found the material on the changing roles of women and how they were reflected in dress and makeup fascinating, and I wanted more of this. I also found the rise of women's occupational choices related to the beauty industry interesting. But, I did not think it necessarily "melded" well with the legislative and regulatory material, and the activism was a social phenomenon rather than one focused on women's groups. In all, this is a very well-researched work that provides little bits to a number of different areas of interest, each of which might merit more on their particular focus. Time will tell.

LYNNE M. DUNPHY, PhD, FNP
Assistant Dean, Graduate Program
Christine E. Lynn College of Nursing
Florida Atlantic University
Boca Raton, FL 33431

One Nation Uninsured: Why the U.S. Has No National Health Insurance

By Jill Quadagno

(New York: Oxford University Press, 2005) (274 pages; $28.00 cloth)

Jill Quadagno's timely book is a substantial contribution to the historical scholarship that attempts to explain why the United States has failed to adopt a national health insurance program. *One Nation Uninsured* is opportune because contemporary health care policy experts have voiced concerns about the re-emerging problems of access, cost, and quality in the American health care delivery system. Presently, government statistics estimate that 45 million Americans lack health insurance coverage, despite the fact that the ever-increasing cost of health care in the United States exceeds that of any other industrialized country in the world. Nurses interested in the history of health care policy will find her book both accessible and informative.

Quadagno's central thesis is that health interests – primarily providers, insurers, and employers – successfully blocked adoption of universal health insurance throughout the course of twentieth-century America and only allowed incremental reforms when they have served their own self-interests. Her argument echoes the analysis of other historians in recent years. Colin Gordon's *Dead on Arrival,* [1] for example, provided a similar narrative to explain the lack of national health insurance in the United States.

Chapters 1 and 2 discuss health care politics prior to 1960. This was a period in which organized medicine worked hard to ward off federal intrusion into health care during the Progressive years, fought to ensure that national health care was not included in the Social Security legislation of 1935, and prevented adoption of national health insurance during the Truman years. Meanwhile, the establishment and growth of Blue Cross and Blue Shield, private alternatives to publicly administered health insurance plans, also characterized these years. Health insurance increasingly became an employee benefit, subject to negotiations and collective bargaining between big business and organized labor.

Quadagno then turns to the reform efforts of the 1960s and the subsequent adoption of Medicare and Medicaid in 1965. Reformers hoped the legislation would be a "first step" toward national health insurance, but they ultimately were proved wrong. Opposition by American medicine and hospital organizations did not prevent the passage of Medicare and Medicaid during the Great Society years. But, once these health interests realized that passage of federal legislation was inevitable, they turned their efforts to making sure the legislation was favorable to providers, insurers, and hospital organizations. The federal government allowed generous reimbursement to both hospitals and physicians for care provided to patients under Medicare and Medicaid.

Although Medicare and Medicaid offered health insurance to older adults and the very poor who previously lacked access to care, the legislation proved to be inflationary due to a lack of incentives for providers and hospital organizations to control health care costs. During the 1970s and beyond, subsequent efforts to adopt national health insurance failed, as economic woes and inflation in the 1970s and budgetary politics in the 1980s and beyond served to constrain reformers' dreams that the state might act to expand access to care. At the same time, however, the economic woes beginning in the 1970s resulted in a shrinking private welfare state, with employers decreasing (or altogether eliminating) health benefit provision.

Quadagno's later chapters focus on the federal government's efforts to constrain the costs of Medicare and Medicaid through regulatory changes in the 1980s. Her book also describes the Medicare catastrophic care debacle of the late 1980s and the failure of national health care reform during the early Clinton years. During the latter years of the twentieth century, insurance companies became vociferous opponents of national health insurance. At the same time, private employer-based health insurance and supplemental "Medigap" coverage for Medicare beneficiaries provided a lucrative market for potential profits, serving as a rationale to rally against government-controlled health care.

Nurses will find Quadagno's book relatively easy to read, with interesting anecdotes and informative quotes from politicians, interest groups, and would-be reformers who shaped the health-policy debates throughout the twentieth century. Her analysis is based on a wealth of primary data sources, including papers from the Johnson and Nixon administrations, the National Archives, and the archives of the late Senator Claude Pepper. Her secondary sources also include previous scholarship in the history and politics of American health care policy. Consistent with other recent works on the history of American health policy, Quadagno's political history is void of references to organized nursing and the role nurses played in shaping the debate over national health insurance in twentieth-century America. Her treatment of some of the political giants in this story – such as Lyndon Johnson and Claude Pepper – adopt a somewhat celebratory tone at specific points in her narrative. Nevertheless, nurses interested in the politics of health care reform during the twentieth century and some of the major policy debates surrounding the finance of American health care will find that Quadagno's book is a good beginning to understanding the political and societal forces that shaped the existing hybrid private–public welfare state.

JONATHAN GILBRIDE, MSN, CCRN, FNP
Doctoral Candidate
Barbara Bates Center for the Study of the History of Nursing
University of Pennsylvania
Philadelphia, PA 19104

1. Colin Gordon, *Dead on Arrival: The Politics of Health Care in Twentieth Century America* (Princeton, NJ: Princeton University Press, 2003).
2. Colin Gordon, *Dead on Arrival: The Politics of Health Care in Twentieth Century America* (Princeton, NJ: Princeton University Press, 2003).

Health Security for All: Dreams of Universal Health Care in America

By Alan Derickson

(Baltimore: The Johns Hopkins University Press, 2005) (240 pages; $30.00 paper)

Throughout the twentieth century, there were spirited debates in the United States regarding the appropriate roles of the public and private sectors to provide for the social welfare needs of the nation's citizens. In *Health Security for All: Dreams of Universal Health Care in America*, Alan Derickson builds on the existing literature on failed efforts to pass health insurance legislation to explore the largely overlooked topic of the American public's movement toward and away from universal health access. Unlike another recently published work on the topic, the author moves beyond the study of the policy itself.[1] He traces changes in societal thought about health and illness, the origins of the ideal of universalism, and the interactions between these as the varying schemes to assure universal access was translated into action. In so doing, he explores larger questions of how ideals of health care are created and, in turn, re-created by the cultural, social, economic, and political contexts of the time in which they evolve.

Although little is known about the accessibility of health care services during the nineteenth century, Derickson begins by suggesting that the need for universal health coverage was linked to the emergence of the modern medical marketplace and the subsequent quest to find the "paying patient." He then traces not only how the ideal of universalism was shaped by persistent concerns over the escalating cost of medical care but also societal discourse on the economic and moral worth of individuals and their utility to society. Debates over whether insurance should be compulsory or voluntary, publicly or privately financed, assured through a living wage or state-sponsored health insurance abounded; yet, there was consensus across the political spectrum that *all* Americans should have some form of health security.

Derickson's research reveals that an amazing array of motivations, justifications, and strategies for achieving universal access emerged throughout the twentieth century. For example, in the early 1900s, organized labor fought for a "living wage" rather than compulsory insurance. This approach lost favor during the 1930s when a dance among labor, business, and government set the stage for other voluntary approaches, such as employer-based strategies, to flourish. By the end of the 1940s, health benefits were regularly used as bargaining chips in labor negotiations. Of note, although Derickson highlights the contributions of theologian and economist Father John Ryan to the quest for a "living wage," he overlooks the contributions that "social gospellers" made to the advancement of this cause and to the development of New Deal Era social policy.[2]

Derickson wrote this book, in part, with the hope of offering insights that would strengthen the next generation of reforms. Regardless of the authors' underlying, although not explicitly stated, assumption that universal access is a goal worthy of achieving, his analysis is balanced and the book is well researched. Derickson offers valuable insight into why health reformers were able to shape the policy debate but were not successful in their attempts to determine national policy. Although these reformers' impassioned advocacy for their cause was often a great strength, in some instances, it was a weakness. A thorough analysis of the failed Clinton plan is premature; yet, the author suggests that it was the administration's dedication to all-inclusive universalism, combined with flaws in "policy design and political execution" (p. 162), that marked its demise. The administration's un-wavering dedication to a certain ideal and insistence on broad change were unsuccessful with politicians, and arguably the American public, who typically prefer incremental approaches to policy change. Unlike other twentieth-century innovations, such as the American hospice movement, many reform campaigns have failed due to the inability of elite reformers to mobilize a critical mass of social support to reframe the policy debate. In contrast, hospice advocates achieved passage of the Medicare hospice benefit at unprecedented speed, despite well-reasoned arguments against its passage and a conservative administration eager to rein in the Medicare program.[3] The movement's politically astute leaders were able to propel hospice onto the legislative agenda, but it was the compelling stories of dying patients and their families, as well as a strong message from constituents back home, that tipped the scales of political will in favor of hospice.

In conclusion, the Institute of Medicine recently called for universal health coverage by 2010.[4] Derickson offers a provocative analysis of how and why, in 2006, the United States stands alone as the *only* developed and prosperous nation in the world that has not been able to achieve such coverage. This book is refreshing and is an important contribution to the health-policy literature. It will be of interest to politicians, social scientists, health-policy scholars, historians, and contemporary reformers, regardless of political persuasion.

Joy Buck, PhD, RN
Postdoctoral Fellow
Barbara Bates Center for the Study of the History of Nursing
Center for Health Outcomes & Policy Research
University of Pennsylvania School of Nursing
Philadelphia, PA 19104

1. Rick Mayes, *Universal Coverage: The Elusive Quest for National Health Insurance* (Ann Arbor: University of Michigan Press, 2004).
2. For more information on the Social Gospel movement and American culture, see Susan Curtis, *A Consuming Faith: The Social Gospel and Modern American Culture* (Columbia: University of Missouri Press, 2001).
3. Joy Buck, "Rights of Passage: Reforming Care of the Dying, 1965–1986" (PhD diss., University of Virginia, Charlottesville, 2005).
4. Institute of Medicine, Board on Health Care Services, *IOM Report Calls for Universal Health Coverage by 2010; Offers Principles to Judge, Compare Proposed Solutions*, June 14, 2004, http://www4.nationalacademies.org/news.nsf/isbn/0309091055?OpenDocument.

Nursing Against the Odds: How Health Care Cost Cutting, Media Stereotypes, and Medical Hubris Undermine Nurses and Patient Care

By Suzanne Gordon
(Ithaca, NY: Cornell University Press, 2005) (489 pages; $19.77 cloth)

Are we "*Nursing Against the Odds*"? In her book of this title, Suzanne Gordon offers compelling arguments to support this concept. As a journalist, the author has spent a number of years interviewing and reporting about nursing. She categorizes her book into three main foci: the nurse and doctor relationship, the media and nursing, and health care cost cutting. In so doing, she presents the odds that stack up against the nursing profession. Gordon draws on in-depth interviews of staff nurses, nursing managers, physicians, administrators, and technicians. She includes information from research studies by economists, sociologists, historians, and nursing leaders; and she provides extensive firsthand reporting of observations of health care delivery to help the reader understand today's nursing environment.

Gordon identifies her mantra, "recruitment and retention," as a prime motivating passion for writing this manuscript. After reading her book, however, this reviewer was left feeling saddened at the negative but often true depiction of the nursing profession. Reflecting on the author's message – the support of nursing recruitment – leads one to ponder whether or not an eighteen-year-old person looking at nursing today might seek other career choices after reading *Nursing Against the Odds*.

Gordon clearly describes the dysfunctional relationship between nurses and physicians. She argues that physicians have historically prevented nurses from gaining prestige and have blocked their ability to maintain a direct revenue stream. Stories abound relating to physicians belittling, disrespecting, and openly devaluing the role nurses play in patient care. Indeed, poor communication and lack of physician respect are cited as impacting patient safety in several firsthand stories offered by nurses in Gordon's book.

Nursing Against the Odds also challenges nurses to communicate more effectively with physicians, arguing that nurses need to tell physicians what they do when the doctor is not present. Nurses often fail to take credit for preventing things from going wrong, Gordon argues. She further explores aspects of nursing language that hinder good communication. Nurses' notes, for example, highlight this communication void. One basic question is: Why are physician's not reading nurses notes, even though nurses have important patient care information to share? Her answer: Only nurses understand "nursing language," and this is problematic. Nurses must connect with all members of the medical team to be effective.

Gordon also questions the theoretical caring aspects of nursing by quoting Sioban Nelson, "If you read the caring discourse in nursing closely, you'll find that many theorists of caring actually put down the technical and medical" (p. 139). This "moral reframing," Gordon offers, is done to place nurses on a higher moral ground than physicians. Does this send the message that other members of the medical team are not as caring as nurses? Caring is an important aspect of nursing, but caring without technical skills and medical knowledge could not be called nursing.

Regarding nursing and the media, the author argues that nurses are often the brunt of journalistic humor and are exploited to spice up a plot line. Angel or sex nymph, villain or sweet but dumb, drunkards, and battle-axes are among the character types portraying nurses on screen or in print. Nurses have reacted to television selling a negative portrayal of the nurse role, such as their protests when *ER's* character Abby Lockart solved her frustration with nursing by entering medical school. Many nurses, however, appear ambivalent about publicly supporting and marketing their profession. Indeed, when the media comes knocking on a nurse's door for an interview, nurses demurely respond and often give credit for health care successes to the physician. On a positive note, Gordon counters the negative depictions with examples of media representations of nurses as complex, knowledgeable, and caring humans. She cites Peter Baida's prize-winning *A Nurse's Story*[1] and Anne Perry's contemporary fiction series, *The Face of a Stranger*,[2] among others. Each offered portrayals of nurses who broke away from the traditional media mold.

A disturbing message in *Nursing Against the Odds* is the repeated portrayal that nurses are unable to articulate what they do. Gordon describes nursing as having a "... poor practice narrative," and she describes this as a "worldwide phenomena" (p. 205). Nurses are hesitant and fearful, and they struggle to find the words that define who they are and what they do. True, nursing is not easy to define because nurses must meet the health care needs of a variety of patients in many different situations and settings. If they cannot communicate a clear picture to society of what they do, Gordon offers, it will be difficult to gain the respect of physicians, the payers, their patients, and themselves. A clear message is sent: that nurses, in order to advance their profession, must publicize and take credit for what they do.

Gordon dedicates the largest section of her book to the review of how cost containment efforts have affected nursing. In hospitals, managed care's cost cutting efforts have reduced nursing staffing. Although nurses have faithfully tried to fill the staffing gaps by caring for a greater number of patients, hospitals have started contracting with higher paid, temporary nursing staff when the gaps become dangerous. Gordon explains how managed-care limitations and the restructuring of health care are starting to take its toll. Patients complain of angry, frustrated, and less than caring nurses at their bedside. Some nurses respond to health care change by retreating, while others send a "poor me" message – but there are also those who respond proactively. This book highlights these issues and many others that make for good discussion among students in nursing, history, medicine, and women's studies, all of whom can benefit by reading this book.

Is nursing fighting against insurmountable odds? Nurses entrenched in this profession will realize that Gordon's concerns have validity. However, although the first step toward recovery from any problem involves acknowledging that a problem exists, it is important not to *spread the dread* by solely highlighting nursing's shortcomings. Nurses also need to examine their successes in gaining more power. Gordon's book gains high marks for compiling valid information that addresses the deterrents. Now let us allow equal time to look at what nursing has done and is doing right.

MARCELLA RUTHERFORD, MBA, MSN, RN
Doctoral Student
Florida Atlantic University
Christine E. Lynn School College of Nursing
Director of Operations
Surgical Associates of Palm Beach County
Boca Raton, FL 33431

1. Peter Baida, *A Nurse's Story, and Others* (Jackson: University Press of Mississippi, 2001).
2. Anne Perry, *The Face of a Stranger* (New York: Ballantine Books, 1990).

Autism and the Myth of the Person Alone

By Douglas Biklen with Richard Attfield, Larry Bissonnette, Lucy Blackman, Jamie Burke, Alberto Frugone, Tito Rajarshi Mukhopadhyay, and Sue Rubin (New York: University Press, 2005)

The goal of *Autism and the Myth of the Person Alone* is to debunk the social myth that implicitly links cognition with verbal communication abilities. Douglas Biklen would rather we "presume competence." This book provides numerous opportunities for the reader to question why it has taken us so long to recognize that judgment of competence based on mere superficial interaction is very misleading.

In 1912, Eugene Bleuler, a Swiss psychiatrist, first introduced the term "autism." However, it was not until 1943, when Leo Kanner, a psychiatrist from Johns Hopkins, used the word to describe eleven of his young patients, that "autism" was recognized as a classification of medical interest. Kanner used the Greek term "autos" meaning self, to describe the behavioral similarities of his patients: they all seemed to lack interest in other people.

Today we know that autism is a neurobiological condition with varying degrees of impairment in communication, social interactions, and repetitive behaviors. A lot of recent professional research has employed quantitative methods and has focused on the diagnosis and treatment of autism and other related disorders under the broader classification of Pervasive Developmental Disorders. Epidemiological issues of incidence and prevalence have also been of great concern to the research community in recent years.

The fact that Biklen reports on autism, then, is not groundbreaking. But his selection of coauthors is of great importance. Biklen approaches autism from a very different perspective than the researchers who preceded him on this topic. He employed a qualitative research design for a study he conducted over a period of two years. This global ethnography brought together seven people from around the world. Every one of Biklen's coauthors has been labeled as autistic. Several were also classified as "retarded." But, even with these disability labels, this amazing group of individuals has enjoyed success.

The book begins with an introduction and discussion on methods, in which Biklen explains his process of inductive inquiry and purposeful sampling. This is an unusual perspective in an area in which deductive inquiry is the norm. Chapter 1 frames autism as we know it today and contrasts it to the lives of the individuals sharing their autobiographies. Biklen challenges the reader to look through a new lens to understand the dynamic, human component of autism. He argues that autism has been framed as a social construction not unlike culture and race. Observers make judgments without the benefit of input from the observed.

Chapters 2 through 7 are composed of two parts. The first part of each chapter is an introduction written by Biklen to give us the context based on his interactions with the individual, and the second part is written by a coauthor. In Chapter 2, for example, Sue

Rubin, whom some will remember as the young California woman showcased in the CNN documentary, "Autism Is a World," which Biklen coproduced, gives her commentary on the 1943 writings of Leo Kanner. In Chapter 4, Biklen interviews Tito Rajarshi Mukhopadhyay on topics such as communication, ways of learning, experiences, and his perceptions through the lens of autism. In Chapter 5, Larry Bissonnette expresses his thoughts through remarks on his artwork. Jamie Burke introduces Chapter 8, where he shares a high school essay on his school world. He highlights the fact that teachers orchestrating the school day are a large part of what makes or breaks inclusive education.

In *Autism and the Myth of the Person Alone*, Biklen constructs a fascinating and balanced work consisting of the personal stories of seven individuals for whom the ability to communicate has given them a vehicle with which to give us a glimpse into their innermost thoughts and feelings. Some of the coauthors learned by facilitated communications (FC), a controversial method that teaches those unable to verbally communicate how to type, facilitated by a therapist who directs the student's hand. Other coauthors gained communication skills through tireless work by parents and teachers using a number of pedagogical methods.

Some may look at this work and presume that it is about FC, an area in which Biklen is a specialist; but, that is only a piece of the picture. Advocating for the disabled, in particular those afflicted with autism, is by no means a new role for Biklen, who has been working for and writing about communication issues related to autism since the late 1980s. Educated in history, regional planning, and the social sciences, Biklen is the Dean of the Department of Education at Syracuse University in New York. As founder and Director of the Facilitated Communication Institute at Syracuse since its inception in 1992, Biklen has produced several works to promote the controversial method of communication training.

This book is especially important for historians of science, technology, and medicine because it bridges the gap between knowledge generated about autism through both quantitative and qualitative methods of discovery. In fact, it is a must read for anyone preparing for or even contemplating a career in health care or education. The book could not have come at a better time. As tools for diagnosis of autism have been refined, the number of people diagnosed with the disorder has increased exponentially. It helps readers see life through a lens they may have heretofore deemed unimaginable or, in the case of autism, nonexistent.

Patricia A. White, RN, MSN
Doctoral Student
University of Pennsylvania
School of Nursing
420 Guardian Drive
Philadelphia, PA 19104

First, Do No Harm: Power, Oppression and Violence in Healthcare

Edited by Nancy L. Diekelmann

(Madison: University of Wisconsin Press, 2002) (266 pages, $57.95 cloth; $22.95 paper)

This is an example of a book that is not a historical study, but one that would have been helped if the authors had had some participation by historians. For this reason, a review by an historian of nursing can provide important context. First, to provide some background, the book is an outgrowth of a gathering of scholars at the University of Wisconsin–Madison Nursing Institutes for Heideggerian Hermeneutical Studies. Martin Heidegger, after whom the institute was named, was a major force in the development of existentialism in the first half of the twentieth century. One of the tasks he set for himself was to discover the meaning of being. This required investigation into the tools with which men and women are basically concerned, along with exploration of the basic situation, aims, and moods of humans. Exploring the implications of such an investigation into health and human science is the task that the Madison Institute set out to answer through interpretative phenomenology.

The aim is to give, in this book and in subsequent volumes, an understanding of the sociocultural, personal, and medical constitution of the body and being in health and illness. This is an ambitious task, but one that basically requires some knowledge of how individuals in the past look at these issues. Here, the authors make assumptions, which do not always coincide with what this reviewer has found. Therefore, one of my recommendations for future conferences of the group is to have an interchange with some historians of nursing.

Five articles are included in the book. James J. Fletcher, Mary Cipriano Silva, and Jeanne M. Sorrell author the first, entitled "Harming Patients in the Name of Quality of Life." They are concerned that quality of life is determined too rigidly by the biomedical model of medicine, and, using dementia as an example, they urge the recognition of the humanness of such individuals despite the loss of cognitive functions. The problem is that they put too much of the burden on the health care provider to gain such knowledge when the contact of the professionals with the client is generally limited.

The real difficulty of getting information about qualify of life is emphasized by a case history compiled by Kathryn Hopkins Kavanagh, whose friend and nursing colleague underwent a kidney and pancreas transplant. Kavanagh followed the case closely through nearly one hundred interviews with her friend while she was undergoing this life crisis. The author demonstrates effectively that both she and her friend, as professional nurses, often found themselves helpless to deal with the issues that arose. It is a moving and personalized story in which the patient eventually decides to allow herself to die. Although Kavanagh consoled herself with the words of her friend's father, that dying in this case was healing, she emphasizes the difficulties that even the best intentioned and most devoted individuals have in dealing with the reality of institutionalized care.

Rebecca Sloan conducted interviews with fifty-six patients suffering from end-stage renal disease (ESRD) and fourteen family members. Using interpretive phenomenology as the philosophical background, the author describes and interprets experiences of ESRD and its treatment. She emphasizes the importance of treating each individual patient as a real person with his or her own wants and needs, and how each patient with ESRD also affects family and loved ones. Dialysis units are compared to conditions at major airports, persons arriving and departing from an assigned dialysis chair, with only minutes between "passengers" for technicians and providers to ready equipment for the next treatment. Patients tend to slip into the distance, and when the expected results do not always occur, there is a tendency first to examine the technology rather than the patient. As technology increases, what can the nurse and other medical providers do in a Faustian bargain, which tends to rob the personhood in exchange for biological survival?

Elizabeth Smythe examines the violence of everyday health care with an example of a woman who anticipated but did not go through natural childbirth. She uses Heidegger's concept of the violence of everyday life to explore the subject of the woman and her reactions in considerable detail, as well as those of several others patients whose hospitalizations did not proceed as anticipated. For the purpose of her analysis, Smythe deliberately sought out what she considered violence that is often hidden or taken for granted in what we do in everyday practice, "what is in itself uncaring, unthoughtful behavior" (p. 166), in situations that are just part of being a client or a patient. She also emphasizes the importance of the caregiver and quotes Caussin in the *Old English Dictionary*: "The most Sacred things are violenced, and the most Profane are licensed" (p. 200). Professionals who tend to follow the habits and rituals of practice have to stop and consider the violence inherent in many of our standards and procedures.

Claire Burke Draucker and Joanne M. Hessmiller have gathered stories of women who experienced rape and sexual violence. Stories of violence reveal much about the victims. It is also part of reparative therapy for victims to tell their stories as part of a healing experience. The authors emphasize that the health care professional should encourage patients to talk about what happened to them and that the health care professional should listen attentively to them.

In retrospect, most of what the authors in this book say has been said by generations of nurses before them. It is not a new task for health care providers to listen to or be supportive of their patients. What this book does, however, is put this emphasis into what often can only be called scientific jargon. Sometimes efforts to make the articles appear more scientific are carried to the extreme. Whenever a complicated word exists, it is used instead of a simple one. Citations abound to even the most common statement. For example, to indicate that visiting a friend in the hospital is based on concern, hope, and friendship does not, in my mind, call for three separate citations. Still the book has an important message, one with which most nurses would agree. It recommends practices that we learned as students, but it is good to have the message reinforced; and we can now say that what we have long been taught to do is being validated by ongoing research.

Vern L. Bullough, PhD, DSci, RN (Retired)
State University of New York Distinguished Professor Emeritus
Center for Sex Research at California State University
Northridge Department of Nursing
University of Southern California
Lake Village, CA 91324

NEW DISSERTATIONS

Compiled for the *Nursing History Review* by Jonathan Erlen, PhD, History of Medicine Librarian, Health Science Library System, and Assistant Professor, Graduate School of Public Health at the University of Pittsburgh, Pittsburgh, Pennsylvania.

Catherine Boyce, "Parenting Advice to Immigrants, 1889–1916: Settlement House Leaders and Kindergartners," PhD dissertation, The University of Chicago, Chicago, IL.
> *Pub No*: 3168323
> *ISBN*: 0-542-04082-4
> *Source*: DAI-A 66/03, p. 1161, Sep 2005

This study examined the tension between helping immigrant families maintain their cultural heritage and helping them assimilate – as reflected in parenting advice. All of the parenting advice, to some extent or another, reflected the belief that both the nation and the immigrants themselves would be best served if immigrant families assimilated as much as possible into the majority culture. The more flexible the leaders were in applying a diversity of educational ideologies and assimilation models, the better able they were to address the native culture of those receiving their parenting advice.

Katherine Joy Buck, "Rights of Passage: Reforming Care of the Dying, 1965–1986," PhD dissertation, University of Virginia, Charlottesville, VA.
> *Pub No*: 3169641
> *ISBN*: 0-542-05736-0
> *Source*: DAI-B 66/03, p. 1389, Sep 2005

This study examines the transitions in care for the dying and the processes of developing an alternative to hospital-based care of the dying during the latter half of the twentieth century. In doing so, it examines the juxtaposition of societal attitudes, technology, professional paradigms, and political influence on the evolution of care for the dying in the United States. Specifically, the initiation and development of the hospice movement in the state of Connecticut from 1965 to 1986 was used as a case study to examine the translation of the hospice philosophy of care into a reimbursable model of care under Medicare.

Sharon Fish Mooney, "Worldviews in Conflict: A Historical and Sociological Analysis of the Controversy Surrounding Therapeutic Touch in Nursing," PhD dissertation, University of Rochester, Rochester, NY.

Pub No: 3166442
ISBN: 0-542-01790-3
Source: DAI-B 66/03, p. 1398, Sep 2005

This study argues that the controversy concerning Therapeutic Touch (TT) is primarily related to a clash of worldviews or sets of assumptions held about the nature of reality. The practice of TT appears to hold out the hope of a monistic solution and a harmonial answer to the fragmentation of personhood in a world of expanding medical technology and also appears to provide a uniquely sanctioned role to female empowerment.

Sharon G. Auker, "The Image of the Profession of Nursing and Its Discursive Representation in Print Media," PhD dissertation, The Pennsylvania State University, University Park, PA.

Pub No: 3157516
ISBN: 0-496-89887-6
Source: DAI-B 65/12, p. 6287, Jun 2005

This dissertation examines the image of nursing and the profession of nursing as portrayed in print media and the related implications for nursing retention, recruitment, and, in turn, the nursing shortage. The findings show that the image of a profession is affected by the public's level of knowledge about the profession, the current conditions under which the profession practices, and the portrayal of the group by the mass media.

Carolyn Peoples Veiga, "Case Studies of Resilient Returning Women of African Descent in an RN to BSN Completion Program at an Historically Black College/University: Personal and Academic Lived Experiences," PhD dissertation, University of Maryland, College Park, MD.

Pub No: 3153131
ISBN: 0-496-13650-X
Source: DAI-B 65/11, p. 6073, May 2005

This research constructs a comprehensive description of the personal and academic lived experiences of adult women of African descent who had been identified by the Nurse Entrance Test (NET) as educationally at risk for failure to complete a Bachelor of Science in Nursing degree at a mid-Atlantic historically black college/university. The negotiation of continual challenges allowed these resilient women to persist and to overcome the negative NET prediction: these women had learned through numerous life experiences to reject such negative feedback and believed that with sufficient effort, their educational goals could be and were attained.

Sandra L. Larson, "The Influence of Professions on the Development and Outcome of Federal Regulations That Affect Their Work," PhD dissertation, University of Illinois at Chicago.

Pub No: 3154461
ISBN: 0-496-14900-8
Source: DAI-A 65/11, p. 4334, May 2005

This case study examined the lobbying of the American Association of Nurse Anesthetists and the American Society of Anesthesiologists on the rule-making process of a Health Care Finance Administration (HCFA) rule deferring to states on the issue of physician supervision of nurse anesthetists. The findings show that HCFA's final rule to remove physician supervision of nurse anesthetists is more accurately characterized as a fair and dispassionate analysis of the policy issue as opposed to political favoritism.

Sherrill L. Leifer, "'Prefers Assignments Which Are Creative in Nature': Harriet H. Werley, Army Nurse Corps Leader, 1941–1964," PhD dissertation, University of Wisconsin – Milwaukee.

Pub No: 3154294
ISBN: 0-496-14849-4
Source: DAI-B 65/11, p. 5633, May 2005

This study analyzes Werley's early life, experiences, and contributions to nursing. Werley's experiences, accomplishments, and the impact of her Army career from 1941 to 1964 are highlighted. This historical study of biographical data about a nursing leader adds to the body of knowledge about the phenomenon of leadership. It provided further knowledge about how to create change and achieve success despite challenging obstacles.

Catherine S. Parzynski, "Maternal Medicine: Changing Perceptions of Women's Place in Medicine, Settlement to 1860," PhD dissertation, Lehigh University, Lehigh, PA.

Pub No: 3154562
ISBN: 0-496-14977-6
Source: DAI-A 65/11, p. 4324, May 2005

This study argues that over time, women did not disappear from healing, rather they redefined their place in medicine. American women willingly modified their traditional roles as helpmates and healers and became, instead, practitioners of maternal medicine.

Marsha Jo Sternard, "The Image of the Female Nurse in Medical Dramas, Non-Medical Dramas, Situation Comedies, Made-for-TV Movies, and Made-for-Theatre Movies Shown on Television from 1985–2000," PhD dissertation, University of Wisconsin – Milwaukee.
Pub No: 3154309
ISBN: 0-496-14864-8
Source: DAI-A 65/11, p. 4073, May 2005

This study examined the image of the female nurse from different races, cultures, and ethnic backgrounds on television from 1985 to 2000. The nurses' portrayal was found to have changed little from prior work in the twentieth century.

Lori Guenthner Stinson, "An Exploration of Native Nurse Leadership: Stories of the People," PhD dissertation, The University of Idaho, Moscow, Idaho.
Pub No: 3127613
ISBN: 0-496-74877-3
Source: DAI-A 65/03, p. 1010, Sep 2004

This qualitative study examines the experiences of four Native nurse leaders in order to more fully understand the concept of leadership from their unique perspectives, including experiences of vision, power, humility, and comfort with the title of leader.

Cynthia Toman, "'Officers and Ladies': Canadian Nursing Sisters, Women's Work, and the Second World War," PhD dissertation, The University of Ottawa, Ottawa, Ontario, Canada.
Pub No: NQ85385
ISBN: 0-612-85385-3
Source: DAI-A 64/10, p. 3804, Apr 2004

This research examines Canadian military nurses' work through the lens of medical technology and discourse analysis. War enabled the transformation of at least 4,381 civilian nurses into Canadian Nursing Sisters who served "for the duration." Toman argues that medical technology, gender, and war situated the Nursing Sisters as an expandable and expendable feminine workforce for the military, legitimated their presence at the frontlines of both war and medical technology, and facilitated the formation of a symbolic community and a social memory as military nurses.

Gloria R. Smith, "Liberation Through a Professional Association: A Case Study of the National Black Nurses' Association," PhD dissertation, Union Institute and University, Cincinnati, OH.
Pub No: DP11149
Source: DAI-A 65/07, p. 2792, Jan 2005

This study explores how black nurses responded to the impotence of the nursing profession by adopting the empowerment strategy of organizing around ethnic identity. A sequence of events has been reconstructed because there is no written history of the National Black Nurses' Association (NBNA); and the author has been both a participant and observer. This study suggests that the NBNA has been a failure in achieving radical change but a success in projecting its members into national prominence.

Edward J. Donahue, "The History of the Sacred Heart Hospital School of Nursing, Allentown, Pennsylvania," PhD dissertation, Capella University.
Pub No: 3151315
ISBN: 0-496-11312-7
Source: DAI-A 65/10, p. 3716, Apr 2005

The Sacred Heart Hospital School of Nursing was founded as the educational arm of the Sacred Heart Hospital in Allentown, Pennsylvania. Today, the Sacred Heart Hospital survives but the Sacred Heart Hospital School of Nursing does not. Contained herein are the details of the history of the Sacred Heart Hospital School of Nursing from an antiquarian perspective.

Marguerite Felix Bortolotti, "The Political Economy of Nursing in the Industrialized World: Impacts of Caring, Professionalism and State Policy on the Everyday Practice of Nurses," PhD dissertation, Carleton University, Ottawa, Ontario, Canada.
Pub No: NQ94196
ISBN: 0-612-94196-5
Source: DAI-A 65/09, p. 3574, Mar 2005

This thesis examines the impacts of caring, professionalism, and state policy on the everyday practice of nurses in Canada, France, England, and Italy under policy-reform strategies of cost containment. It argues that there are inherent contradictions built into the different assumptions of the concepts of caring and professionalism, as well as the conditions in which both concepts are engendered.

Carole Shimko Senter, "The American Nurses Association 1965 Position on Education for Nursing: A Policy Study Based on Discourse Analysis," PhD dissertation, The University of Pittsburgh, Pittsburgh, PA.
Pub No: 3149989
ISBN: 0-496-09601-X
Source: DAI-A 65/10, p. 3722, Apr 2005

This nonexperimental case study uses discourse analysis as a means of identifying stakeholders in the nursing education debate and as a method of deconstructing their arguments. This study analyzes one of the most cited documents in nursing history in a new way and presents a new model for policy study based on discourse analysis.

Jayne Elliott, "'Keep the Flag Flying': Medical Outposts and the Red Cross in Northern Ontario, 1922–1984," PhD dissertation, Queen's University at Kingston, Canada.
Pub No: NQ99941
ISBN: 0-612-99941-6
Source: DAI-A 66/02, p. 722, Aug 2005

Following World War I, the Canadian Red Cross established medical outposts in remote areas. This study examines the Ontario Division, which administered the most complex of these outpost programs. The nurses who staffed the small hospitals and nursing stations were essential to the ability of the division to carry out its mission. They were often professionally isolated and inadequately trained for the situations that confronted them, but many derived satisfaction from the adventure, as well as autonomy, friendships, and status.

Carol Lea Whiteside, "The Sources and Forms of Power Used by Florence Nightingale as Depicted in Her Letters Written July 1, 1853 to August 7, 1856," PhD dissertation, Gonzaga University, Spokane, WA.
Pub No: 3162855
ISBN: 0-496-98661-9
Source: DAI-B 66/02, p. 822, Aug 2005

This study examined the letters Nightingale wrote while she served as the Superintendent at the Institute for Ill Gentlewomen in London and during her years serving in the Crimean War. By far, the two most prevalent types of power used by Nightingale were persuasion and authority. With family members and friends, Nightingale used persuasion as a form of power. However, writing to colleagues or the War Office, Nightingale used competent or legitimate authority as the predominant form of power.

OUR SHARED LEGACY

Nursing Education at Johns Hopkins, 1889–2006

EDITED BY MAME WARREN

IN ASSOCIATION WITH THE JOHNS HOPKINS NURSES' ALUMNI ASSOCIATION

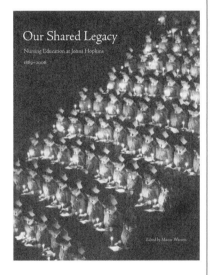

"Conscious of the past, equal to the present, and reaching forward into the future—that's the Hopkins way. That's our shared legacy. That's the challenge of your tomorrow."

With these words to the class of 1988, Barbara Donaho (1956) underscored the complex history of nursing education at Johns Hopkins. From the founding of the hospital's training nursing school in 1889, through years of struggle to achieve full academic recognition as the Johns Hopkins University School of Nursing, Hopkins nurses have maintained high standards of excellence, professionalism, and vigilance—both at the bedside and in the highest realms of leadership.

In this beautifully illustrated volume, the voices of generations of Hopkins nurses combine with a well-researched historical narrative to offer a stirring tribute to Hopkins nursing students and alumni along with unique insight into the history of an admirable and challenging profession.

320 pages, 359 illustrations, $50.00 hardcover

THE JOHNS HOPKINS UNIVERSITY PRESS
1-800-537-5487 • www.press.jhu.edu

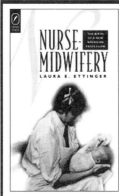

Nurse-Midwifery
The Birth of a New American Profession
Laura E. Ettinger

During the twentieth century modern births in America came to involve mostly male physicians, hospitals, technological interventions, and quick, routine procedures. In a unique and detailed historical study, this first book-length documentation describes the emergence of American nurse-midwifery. In *Nurse-Midwifery*, Ettinger shows how nurse-midwives in New York City; eastern Kentucky; Santa Fe, New Mexico; and other places both rebelled against and served as agents of a nationwide professionalization of doctors and medicalization of childbirth. *Nurse-Midwifery* reveals the limitations that nurses, physicians, and nurse-midwives placed on the profession of nurse-midwifery from the outset because of the professional interests of nursing and medicine. The book argues that nurse-midwives challenged what scholars have called the "male medical model" of childbirth, but the cost of the compromises they made to survive was that nurse-midwifery did not become the kind of independent, autonomous profession it might have been.

$26.95 paper 0-8142-5150-1 $74.95 cloth 0-8142-1023-6 $9.95 CD 0-8142-9100-7

Women, Gender, and Health
Susan L. Smith and Nancy Tomes, Series Editors

THE OHIO STATE UNIVERSITY PRESS
www.ohiostatepress.org   800-621-2736